Do lockdowns and border closures serve the "greater good"?

A cost-benefit analysis of Australia's reaction to COVID-19

Gigi Foster

Professor of Economics, UNSW Business School, University of New South Wales, Sydney, Australia

with Sanjeev Sabhlok

Connor Court Publishing Pty Ltd

Published in 2022 by Connor Court Publishing Pty Ltd.

Connor Court Publishing Pty Ltd
PO Box 7257
Redland Bay QLD 4165
sales@connorcourt.com
www.connorcourt.com

ISBN: 9281922815217

Cover Design by Maria Giordano

Printed in Australia.

Front Cover Photo: Bourke Street Mall during the lockdowns, Wikipedia Commons.

In the past six months we have witnessed a mass worldwide sacrificial event driven by a fear of the unknown and essentially an abandonment of post-Enlightenment thinking. We have been swept up in hysteria and the fanaticism of crowds. Our economy has been stabbed in the stomach.

– Testimony of Gigi Foster to the PAEC, Victoria, August 2020

There is no doubt in my mind, that when we come to look back on this, the damage done by lockdown[s] will exceed any saving of lives by a huge factor.

– Michael Levitt, Nobel Prize winner in Chemistry

Since lockdowns are now known to have had no clear beneficial effect on the number of Covid cases or deaths, there is no trade-off to be analysed in the area of lockdown policies. There is just loss all around.

– Paul Frijters et al in The Great Covid Panic

It is possible that lockdown[s] will go down as one of the greatest peacetime policy failures in modern history.

– Douglas Allen, Professor of Economics at Simon Fraser University

Contents

CONTENTS

Preface

Rational public policymaking considers both sides of any proposed policy: benefits and costs. When the costs of lockdown policy have been raised during the COVID era, people have sometimes assumed that those costs are about "just the economy," implying that "the economy" is something separable from human health. Yet there are health and longevity costs of lockdowns, apart from their short-run impacts on normal economic and social functioning, quality of life, and general well-being.

In the first half of 2020, the costs of locking down economies should have been weighed against the projected benefits. Best guesses needed to be made about the areas of human well-being directly and indirectly affected by lockdown policies. Among other things, we needed to consider the loss of happiness due to loneliness from social isolation, the crowding-out of healthcare for problems other than COVID, the long-term costs to our children and university students of disrupted education, and the economic losses of shuttered businesses, increased inequality, and crowded-out government spending in future years.

In August 2020, I prepared a draft cost-benefit analysis (CBA) for consideration by the Victorian State Parliament[i] that was an illustration of how such an exercise could be conducted by the government, whose responsibility it was to provide a rational justification for the Victorian lockdown policies.

This report updates my outline CBA of August 2020. It includes more context about the methods and about how to approach the robust policy deliberation process that Australian governments should have undertaken early in 2020. It is structured like a standard CBA

---

[i] Public Accounts and Estimates Committee (PAEC) of the Victorian Parliament, *Inquiry into the Victorian Government's Response to the Covid-19 Pandemic*, 12 August 2020, https://bit.ly/3MEvwj8.

except that I do not analyse multiple options. I consider only one: the actual policies adopted in Australia. The alternative that I consider – the benchmark against which the impact of lockdowns is compared – is for the government to have put in place policies that delivered outcomes similar to what Sweden or other "risk-based-restrictions" countries experienced.

Sourcing the data needed for such a process continues to be a challenge, but this is not new, and it is a challenge that economists are trained to meet. We try, using the best data available, to come up with reasonable estimates. It would have been nice, for example, to have access to more reliable and up-to-date Australian data about various aspects of human well-being and suffering. While tools like ANUPoll are useful, we need to build even better tools for the analysis of human welfare in Australia. Using conservative assumptions on many different categories of costs and generous assumptions about the benefits of lockdowns, I have pieced together an estimate.

It is in Australia's interests to provide access to better quality data about its people, activities, and society, so that we can learn more about how to protect and promote welfare. To achieve this, Australia's government departments and research institutions must develop more robust, up-to-date, and relevant data sources and make them accessible not only to policymakers with a duty to evaluate their policies, but also to independent researchers and the broader public.

I would like to thank Paul Frijters and Michael Baker for their comments on early drafts of this document. Their input greatly helped me to refine the structure and assumptions used. I am also grateful to UNSW's Health@Business network that provided modest funding for research to support this project.

My deepest heartfelt gratitude goes to Sanjeev Sabhlok, who drew together most of the initial content of this document from existing sources, added and adjusted content diligently at my request, and has been a tireless supporter of the endeavour.

I use the terms COVID and COVID-19 interchangeably in this document. I do not, however, revise the usage in published sources. The disease is increasingly being shortened in the literature to simply "covid."

Gigi Foster

Sydney, 1 August 2022

1. Executive Summary

The world has been shaken by the response of governments to the COVID-19 pandemic in a way unlike what we have seen in any prior global health event. What started as a local health anomaly in one Chinese province quickly became a world-stopping crisis affecting every major nation in 2020. Industries from travel to manufacturing suffered sudden, acute disruptions due to political action to lock down cities and block the free movement of people and goods within and between countries. Was all of this necessary to save lives, or did it on net produce human damage?

This report aims to evaluate whether Australia's COVID lockdown policies – a central feature of our COVID policy response – were on net helpful or harmful. The report is divided into two parts, of which the first is a background discussion that contextualises the analysis, and the second part estimates the costs and benefits of the Australian COVID lockdowns.

1.1 Part 1: Background

I start by discussing the characteristics of good policy processes and summarising the information known early in 2020 that was relevant to responding to COVID. The magnitude of the pandemic is also discussed by reference to history.

1.1.1 *What was known pre-COVID*

On 24 January 2020, at the beginning of the Wuhan lockdowns, Gauden Galea – the World Health Organisation (WHO)'s representative in China – said that "trying to contain a city of 11 million people is new to science. The lockdown of 11 million people is unprecedented in public health history, so it is certainly not a recommendation the WHO has made."[1] This statement summarises the WHO's known

---

[1] Senger, Michael P. (2020). "China's Global Lockdown Propaganda Campaign," in *Tablet*, 16 September 2020. https://bit.ly/3yS93eD.

position on the wisdom of lockdowns in 2019, including its official guidance on managing flu-like pandemics, and was also reflected in official policy positions of the developed world before the arrival of COVID-19.

Years before COVID's arrival, the late Donald Henderson, a major figure in epidemiology who was instrumental in eradicating small-pox from the planet, opined that it is impossible to stop most viruses through border control.[2] Henderson contended that the spread of most viruses cannot be stopped unless the first case (the "index case") in a country is stopped, and the next such "first" case is stopped, and every additional index case is stopped as it erupts. He noted that some viruses can indeed be controlled through quarantines of the sick, and successful attempts have been made to do so (e.g., for Ebo-la). For most viruses, including the flu, he argued that if even a single person who may not have obvious symptoms slips through the net of control, then the battle is lost. It is far more sensible in such cases, Henderson argued, not to implement hard border controls but rather to manage the disease in order to minimise harm. In his words: "this idea that in this day and age one is going to intercept people coming across the border and you're going to stop the spread of the disease is a concept that was antiquated a very long time ago."[3]

Extended lockdowns of whole populations had never been used in the history of pre-COVID disease control and were regarded as unwise by eminent epidemiological experts. They were known to cause significant negative effects on many other dimensions of society, including our ability to continue to control the target disease.[4]

---

[2] See Donald Henderson's comments on this topic from timestamp 32:35 on a panel at the 5 March 2010 conference on "The 2009 H1N1 experience: policy implications for future infectious disease emergencies," at http://youtu.be/8rEV857R0LE (Role of Disease Containment in Control of Epidemics (Panel)).

[3] See from timestamp 33:55 onwards at http://youtu.be/8rEV857R0LE.

[4] See the discussion of Donald Henderson's position and the history of the use of lock-downs provided by Jay Bhattacharya here: https://youtu.be/Cfjcr55XgC0 ("Unscientific over-reaction to COVID & the correct way to deal with it - Jay Bhattacharya of Stanford"), and the following analysis and re-print of a paper by Henderson (Disease Mitigation Measures in the Control of Pandemic Influenza, in *Biosecurity and Bioterrorism: Biodefense Strategy, Practice, and Science*; Volume 4, Number 4, 2006) here: https://archive.ph/0SQx9.

Further, counterintuitive though it may seem, there are arguably great public health benefits from human inter-mingling. Some of these may derive directly from our interaction with pathogens, including when we travel internationally. Since at least her "Princeton in Europe" lecture of 2013, Dr Sunetra Gupta of Oxford University has argued that global immunity to viruses is strengthened from international travel:

> Virulent pathogens cannot be the only things we bring back from countries where they've originated. It is more likely that we're constantly importing less virulent forms which go undetected because they're asymptomatic and these may well have the effect of attenuating the severity of infection with their more virulent cousins.
>
> After all, the oldest trick up our sleeves is, as vaccination goes, is to use a milder species to protect against a more virulent species. Perhaps this is something we're inadvertently achieving by mixing more widely with a variety of international pathogens.[5]

According to Dr Gupta, the same principle applies to children, who "benefit from being exposed to this (COVID) and other seasonal coronaviruses."[6] The logic is that getting a less harmful infection protects children against more serious infections in the future. Therefore, Dr Gupta contends, "the best way to [safeguard against pandemics] is to build up a global wall of immunity. And it may be that we're unwittingly achieving this through our current patterns of international travel." As part of our response to COVID-19, we have paused this potential mechanism of building group-level immunity to pathogens.

The WHO's position on pandemic management prior to COVID-19 included recommending some voluntary preventative measures for a virus like COVID, such as handwashing and avoiding

---

[5] http://youtu.be/kclL0F985DY ("Sunetra Gupta showed in 2013 how international travel eliminates the prospect of A major pandemic").

[6] *Evening Standard* (2020). "The Londoner: Let children be exposed to viruses, says Professor Gupta," 2 September 2020, https://bit.ly/3MB2vVy.

crowds, but no border closures and quarantines, and no mandated restrictions on the movement of healthy people under any circumstances.[7] If such restrictions had been favoured by pre-COVID scientific consensus, this would have been reflected in many scientific contributions prior to 2020, and governments' official pandemic plans, advocating policies like lockdowns after evaluating their costs and benefits. In fact, to my knowledge, virtually no scholarly works published after WWII and prior to 2020 argue that restrictions on the movements of healthy populations would result or ever have resulted in positive net benefits in terms of human welfare, well-being, or lives.[8]

1.1.2 COVID in historical context

A key element of contextualising a cost-benefit analysis of any policy is to understand the magnitude of the problem that the policy purports to address. It has been known since early 2020 that the threat posed by COVID is not severe by historical or pathogenic comparison. Victoria's pandemic plan of 10 March 2020 contained the statement that (the original strain of) "COVID-19 is assessed as being of moderate clinical severity."[9] It has also been clear since 17 February 2020 that COVID is largely a non-event in children but can be severe in the elderly and those with comorbidities.[10] Accordingly, the Vic-

---

[7] See the WHO's pre-COVID (October 2019) report ("Non-pharmaceutical public health measures for mitigating the risk and impact of epidemic and pandemic influenza"), together with the annexure that provides detailed scientific backing for the WHO's recommendations: https://bit.ly/3yO2No9 (Report); https://bit.ly/3yQVETX (Annexure).

[8] The sole exception of which I am aware is the following work, which envisions a pathogenic threat far worse than COVID: Boyd, Matt et al (2018). "Economic evaluation of border closure for a generic severe pandemic threat using New Zealand Treasury methods," in *Australian and New Zealand Journal of Public Health*, vol. 42 no. 5, https://bit.ly/3NvMMaj.

[9] The Victorian Government's "COVID-19 Pandemic Plan for the Victorian Health Sector," dated 10 March 2020, is no longer available from the Victorian Government's original website (https://bit.ly/3G61X7C), but a copy of the report is available at https://bit.ly/3wJEnti.

[10] *China CDC Weekly* (2020). "Vital Surveillances: The Epidemiological Characteristics of an Outbreak of 2019 Novel Coronavirus Diseases (COVID-19) – China, 2020," 2(8): 113-122, https://bit.ly/3cSQCNY, 17 February 2020. For example, the paper reports that "The ≥80 age group had the highest case fatality rate of all age groups at 14.8%." This

torian pandemic plan of early March 2020 "[f]ocused on protecting vulnerable Victorians, including with underlying health conditions, compromised immune systems, the elderly, Aboriginal and Torres Strait Islanders, and those from culturally and linguistically diverse communities." This statement bears a striking resemblance to the advice of the much-maligned Great Barrington Declaration of October 2020.[11]

According to the United States Centers for Disease Control and Prevention (the CDC), there were at least 50 million global deaths[12] in 1918-1919 from the Spanish flu, when the world's population was 1.8 billion. The current world population is 7.9 billion, meaning that around 219 million people would need to die of COVID if the COVID pandemic were in the league of the Spanish flu in terms of raw numbers of deaths. As displayed in Figure 1.1, about 6.3 million COVID deaths were reported by Worldometer[13] by 27 May 2022, or more than 30 times fewer than 219 million.

On 9 April 2022, John Ioannidis of Stanford, one of the world's most highly citied epidemiologists today, wrote to Sanjeev Sabhlok: "You are correct, the 1918 flu was 50-500 times worse than COVID-19 once you adjust for population size and for age distribution. I have highlighted this recently in a paper on the end of the pandemic that includes a detailed table comparing the impact of pandemics versus the seasonal flu. Deaths from SARS-CoV-2 COVID-19 was just 1.5-4 times the equivalent of three seasons of seasonal flu (most likely closer to the 1.5 number actually). Spanish flu was 100-1000 times bigger than 3 seasons of seasonal flu https://onlinelibrary.wiley.com/doi/10.1111/eci.13782".[14] Augmenting this conclusion is the fact that since the Spanish flu severely

---

information was widely known by March 2020 in expert circles, which led to the recognition in the Victorian pandemic plan of the age distribution of COVID risk, along with the overall moderate clinical severity of the disease.

[11] Great Barrington Declaration, 4 October 2020, https://archive.ph/CrP2z.

[12] Centers for Disease Control and Prevention, "1918 Pandemic (H1N1 virus)" – website as at 20 May 2022 (https://bit.ly/3Lvztp2).

[13] https://www.worldometers.info/coronavirus/.

[14] Email from John Ioannidis to Sanjeev Sabhlok dated 9 April 2022: https://bit.ly/3NAhK1h.

Comparing four pandemics

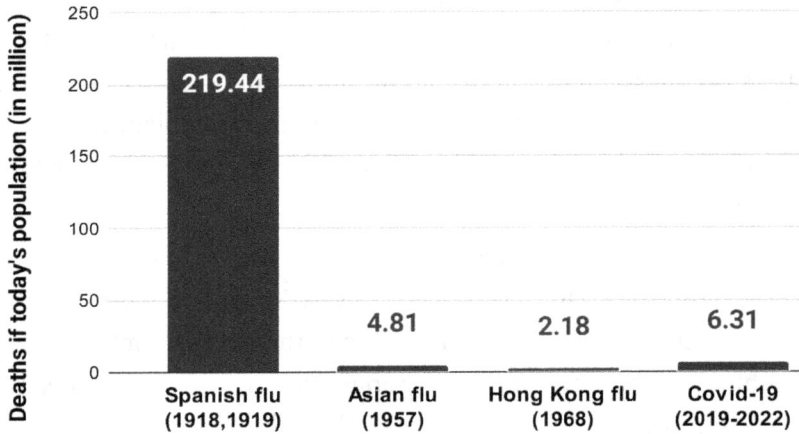

Figure 1.1: A comparison of the relative magnitude of four pandemics[15]

impacted the young, while COVID's victims are mainly elderly, the Spanish flu was even more lethal in terms of potential life years lost.

Even if the many legitimate questions about COVID death reporting are ignored, the severity of the COVID pandemic is in the range of the Asian flu of 1957 (also shown in Figure 1.1), in response to which healthy populations were not locked down.

1.1.3 *Providing a cost-benefit analysis is the responsibility of the government*

It is incumbent upon a democratic government pursuing sound policy-making principles to conduct and provide for public examination a cost-benefit analysis (CBA) of major policies that transparently estimates and weighs all known or expected benefits and all known or expected harms of the policies. Prior to COVID, there was bipartisan support for the following tests to be satisfied in order for a policy to pass: (a) a test of liberty (i.e., the government must not interfere in people's life without a strong justification); and (b) a test of reason (i.e., the justification so provided must be evidence-based and

---

[15] Data as at 10 May 2022. Source spreadsheet: https://archive.ph/wAh2Q. Data for the spreadsheet drawn from sources described here: https://bit.ly/3sKGyvt.

transparent). These two tests are operationalised through conducting a CBA, an approach to policy evaluation that is deeply embedded within Australia's policy processes. However, no such analysis has been released to justify COVID lockdowns.

On 12 August 2020, in light of the government's failure to discharge its responsibility in this regard, I presented a preliminary CBA of Victoria's lockdowns to the Public Accounts and Estimates Committee of Victoria's State Parliament.[16] My analysis was intended as a demonstration of approach and offered a generous estimate of the benefits and only a partial accounting of the costs of lockdowns. I noted that a comprehensive CBA would need to factor in a wide variety of additional costs, many of which I enumerated but did not fully cost out in the document.

No level of Australian government has yet provided a CBA justifying COVID lockdowns. The present report expands my August 2020 draft CBA by providing estimates for more cost and benefit categories, and updates it to cover the costs and plausible benefits of COVID lockdown policies implemented through the end of 2021.

1.2 Part II: The cost-benefit analysis

This expanded CBA confirms that the costs of wholesale lockdowns for Australia are far greater than their benefits in a COVID world, even using the most conservative assumptions in favour of the government's lockdown policies.

1.2.1 *Methodological observations*

A few methodological observations are in order.[17]

This CBA is retrospective, not prospective.

A proper policy analysis using a CBA approach considers not just one policy alternative (lockdowns, in this case) but a wide range of

---

[16] Public Accounts and Estimates Committee (PAEC) of the Victorian Parliament, *Inquiry into the Victorian Government's Response to the Covid-19 Pandemic*, 12 August 2020, https://bit.ly/3MEvwj8.

[17] I am indebted to Sanjeev Sabhlok, former Victorian Treasury economist, for providing much of the information in this report to do with the typical usage of CBA within Australian governments.

options. A scenario analysis is also usually included to accommodate the inevitable uncertainty about projected costs and benefits. Only then is the appropriate policy selected. While this report alludes to a range of potential options that were available to the government at the outset of the pandemic, it is retrospective and looks only at the effects of the actual policies that have been implemented in Australia, relative to a default policy of managing COVID in what would have been considered the best-practice manner before March 2020: i.e., compliance of Australian governments with their own risk-based pandemic plans which preclude wholesale lockdowns or border closures, but include targeted restrictions and voluntary social distancing. Such an approach is proxied in this paper by taking actions that would have delivered outcomes similar to what was seen in countries with policy settings akin to Sweden's in 2020 and 2021.

CBAs are about social welfare, not money.

There is a prevalent misconception that CBAs are about money. They are in fact about social welfare. The approach taken in this report considers statistical lives lost now and in the future, and also counts, for example, the mental health suffering that people endure when they are locked inside their homes. In the CBA presented here, the human welfare costs of lockdowns are put into a currency (quality-adjusted life years, or QALYs) that is used to enumerate estimates for both the costs and the benefits of lockdowns. I also use the newly created WELLBY (well-being year) measure to capture some lockdown costs. Since one year of average healthy life (1 QALY) equates to 6 WELLBYs experienced by a person for one year, this allows suffering across the society to be compared with benefits in the same welfare "currency."

A conservative approach is adopted.

Every assumption about the costs of lockdowns that I make in this CBA is supported directly or indirectly by research literature and evidence.[18]

---

[18] To ensure that the short form/archival URLs can be traced back by future researchers to their original sources even if the archival websites were to shut down, most of them are listed at: https://bit.ly/3cB1507.

The only assumptions I make that have scant backing are my conservative assumptions in favour of lockdowns – i.e., in favour of finding that lockdowns are helpful. I assume in particular that COVID deaths would be avoided (or, more accurately, postponed) by lockdowns. This is an assumption not borne out in other countries' experiences,[19] but arguably true to a small extent in Australia, at least insofar as blocking international travel will have reduced the amount of virus circulating within Australia for a period of time.

Sweden and other countries with targeted restrictions serve as counterfactuals.

To estimate the losses avoided by lockdowns, I consider two alternative counterfactuals: the outcomes achieved by Sweden, and those achieved by a set of six nations with low levels of COVID restrictions. In the final analysis I count the higher of these two estimates – using population-adjusted data from Sweden as the counterfactual – to be the upper-end amount of loss potentially avoided because of Australia's lockdown policies.

Worldometer[20] shows that more than 50 countries with harsh lockdowns have experienced more COVID deaths per million than Sweden which had no lockdowns, mandatory masks, quarantines or border closures. If the Worldometer data is adjusted for Sweden's high latitude (with likely low vitamin D levels), age structure (20% of Sweden's population is over 65 and hence more vulnerable to the virus, compared with 18.9% in the UK and 9.3% across the world), the "dry tinder" effect (a low mortality rate from flu in the December 2019 through March 2020 flu season in Sweden[21] meant that more vulnerable people were around to be attacked by COVID or other

---

[19] E.g., as examined in Herby et al (2022), "A Literature Review and Meta-Analysis of the Effects of Lockdowns on Covid-19 Mortality," SAE/No.200/January 2022, https://bit.ly/3wHaNEP.

[20] https://www.worldometers.info/coronavirus/#countries. As at 3 July 2022, when sorted by COVID deaths per million, 55 countries had a higher COVID death rate than Sweden, including the UK, France, Italy, and the US.

[21] The Public Health Agency of Sweden (2020). "Influenza in Sweden – Season 2019 –2020," Article 20137, 2 October 2020. https://bit.ly/3lvQnJx.

COST-BENEFIT ANALYSIS OF AUSTRALIA'S LOCKDOWNS

respiratory diseases in 2020), higher-density nursing and aged care homes, and likely over-reporting of COVID deaths in Sweden,[22] then the COVID death rate in Sweden would look even more modest. Hence, the choice to use Sweden as a counterfactual likely yields an over-estimate of the benefits of the Australian COVID lockdowns.

1.2.2 Benefits of lockdowns

In this paper I calculate **12,304 deaths** as the upper-end estimate for the number of COVID deaths that could have occurred in Australia during 2020 and 2021 without lockdowns. There were in fact 2,353 COVID deaths in Australia in these two years, even in the presence of lockdowns, so at most **9,951 COVID deaths were avoided by lockdown policies**. On average a COVID death represents a loss of around 5 QALYs,[23] since on average such a death occurs in someone already significantly advanced in age and not in good health.

To this, based on estimates of the incidence and severity of long COVID,[24] one can add 2% of the estimated losses in the form of CO-

---

[22] A 3 August 2021 paper, "Excess mortality due to Covid-19? A comparison of total mortality in 2020 with total mortality in 2016 to 2019 in Germany, Sweden and Spain," by Bernd Kowall et al in *PLoS ONE* (https://bit.ly/3LC5v2D) found that in 2020 Sweden experienced excess mortality of 3%, or around 3,000 extra deaths, which is strikingly low given what one might expect due to the dry tinder effect, but consistent with the estimate by Nobel laureate Michael Levitt of 3%, available at https://bit.ly/38BA0sk. Since 10,000 deaths were reported in Sweden in 2020 as COVID deaths, I deduce that the reported COVID deaths figure is likely a significant over-estimation.

[23] This estimate is based on life tables showing expected QALYs remaining for people with co-morbidities (e.g., https://bit.ly/3wJUyGO) combined with the observation that about 30% of Australia's COVID deaths have occurred in aged care homes, where on entry a resident is expected to have 1 healthy year of life still to live (https://bit.ly/3wKoGll), with the remaining 70% on average still quite old and with 95% probability suffering from one or more co-morbidities (https://bit.ly/3G97oTh). Assuming a generous 6 years of healthy life remaining on average for the 70% of Australian COVID victims residing outside aged care homes, we arrive at 4.5 years of healthy life remaining per average COVID victim, which I then round up to 5 in this report, being generous again.

[24] As detailed in section 8.3.4, in *The Great Covid Panic* my co-authors and I estimated long COVID losses at 5%, but for Australia I use an updated figure of 2%. One reason for this downward adjustment is that we have now had more time to observe the recovery patterns of long COVID cases. The most updated evidence indicates that most of those who do get long COVID are not significantly handicapped in their normal productive activities, and that most cases that would measurably impact life satisfaction resolve within three months and the great majority of the remainder within a year (Hensher,

VID deaths to account for the human cost of long-COVID effects. One can also add an estimated 131 deaths by homicide and traffic accidents, often of people of significantly younger age than the average COVID victim, that would have occurred in a no-lockdown regime.

One therefore arrives at the following upper-end estimate for the total benefit of lockdowns:

9,951 (total COVID deaths averted) x 5 (healthy years lost per COVID death) x 6 (WELLBYs per QALY) x 1.02 (accommodating losses to long COVID) + 131 (non-COVID deaths averted) x 50 (healthy years lost per each such death) x 6 (WELLBYs per QALY) = **343,800** WELLBYs, or **57,300** QALYs, in all.

A further methodological remark: The chronology of restrictions, and monthly cost and benefit accounting

The objective in this report is to consider the incremental benefits and incremental costs of the lockdowns and border closures. To do this I draw on data from the start of lockdowns until the end of December 2021. Full border closures came into effect from 20 March 2020 (https://archive.ph/vYhcs) and lockdowns (stay-at-home orders) from 2 April 2020 in some states.[25] By the end of March 2020 there were around 20 reported COVID deaths in Australia. This figure being negligible, I do not separate out these 20 deaths in the overall analysis. I also assume that border closures and lockdowns impacted any costs and benefits immediately (from 1 April 2020), even though in actuality there would have been some lags. Lockdowns ended in October 2021 in Australia while border closures continued.

An exact approach to estimating the monthly costs and benefits of Australia's lockdown policies would be to divide annual costs and benefits across 9 months in 2020 (April 2020 to December 2020) and

---

Martin et al (2021), "We calculated the impact of 'long COVID' as Australia opens up. Even without Omicron, we're worried," Deakin University, 16 December 2021, https://bit.ly/39JeQs5; Swiss Policy Research, Post Covid Syndrome ("Long Covid"), https://bit.ly/3yVGOeS).

[25] From C6 in the Oxford Covid-19 Government Response Tracker (OxCGRT) database, https://bit.ly/3Bq2ot9.

an appropriate number of months in 2021. For the sake of simplicity, however, the estimates of monthly costs and benefits that I provide in this report assume that there were 12 months of lockdowns/border closures in each of 2020 and 2021. This does not affect the calculations of total costs and benefits, and so any refinements in the future by those inspired to construct more exact monthly costs and benefits would not change the overall conclusion of the analysis.

Dividing the total benefit of 343,800 WELLBYs by 24, we get approximately **14,325 WELLBYs saved per month** during 2020 and 2021 by Australia's stop-start lockdowns and related policies.

How much would Australian society be willing to pay to avoid this quantity of loss?

Taking a high estimate of AU$100,000 as the amount Australian society would be willing to pay to save one QALY – which is an upper-bound estimate based on what the TGA pays in normal years to buy medical interventions that save QALYs[26] – it follows that Australian society would be willing to pay a total of 57,300 (i.e., total QALYs saved) x 100,000 = **AU$5.73 billion** over the course of two years to avoid this magnitude of loss.

The maximum that Australia would normally be willing to spend to prevent an additional **9,951** COVID deaths plus **131** traffic/homicide deaths – even using very conservative assumptions in favour of the government's policies – is therefore around six billion dollars.

In fact, hundreds of billions of dollars have been spent. This itself instantly suggests that alternative policy options should have been considered. This implication is also consistent with the findings of a dollars-and-QALYs-based cost-benefit analysis of Australia's lockdowns published in January 2022 by Martin T. Lally, who finds that at least 11 times more has been spent by the government allegedly to prevent COVID deaths than would have been spent in a normal

---

[26] Estimates taken from: Lally, M. (2022). "A cost–benefit analysis of COVID-19 lockdowns in Australia," in *Monash Bioeth. Rev.*, https://doi.org/10.1007/s40592-021-00148-y.

policy regime, in which Australia would have been willing to spend a maximum of $100,000 per QALY saved.[27]

Have lockdowns avoided 40,000 deaths?

In the lead-up to the election in May 2022, the Prime Minister of Australia is reported to have claimed that 40,000 deaths have been avoided by his "regime" (of lockdowns and border closures).[28] Earlier, he had sent letters to many Australians in which he made a slightly more modest claim of having prevented 30,000 deaths.[29] No substantiating evidence was provided for these assertions, but it is possible that the Prime Minister used estimates based on epidemiological models.

Even if Mr Morrison's most extreme claim were correct and 40,000 COVID deaths had been prevented by lockdowns, that would still bound at **AU$20 billion** the amount Australia would have been willing to pay to pursue the lockdown strategy, using the observation above that Australia is willing to pay at most AU$100,000 per QALY saved. Spending more than that would have diverted scarce resources from other competing priorities that, from a human well-being perspective, also matter.

In fact, we have spent hundreds of billions of dollars pursuing lockdowns and cushioning their economic fallout.

1.2.3 *Costs of lockdowns*

Imposing untargeted crippling restrictions on the vast majority of the population which is not at significant risk from COVID will necessarily cause significant overall harm. Evidence from numerous CBAs undertaken across the world has already indicated, for many countries, that lockdowns are damaging and even that they do not on net save lives.[30]

---

[27] *Ibid.*

[28] *The Guardian* (2022). "Scott Morrison takes credit for saving 40,000 lives from Covid in social media pitch for re-election," 9 April 2022, https://bit.ly/3wCrn9K.

[29] This letter is available in scanned form here: https://bit.ly/3wzQgBW.

[30] E.g., CBAs for the UK (my co-authored book, *The Great Covid Panic*); Australia (Lally, M. (2022). "A cost–benefit analysis of COVID-19 lockdowns in Australia," in *Monash Bioeth. Rev.*, https://doi.org/10.1007/s40592-021-00148-y); and Canada (Allen, Douglas W. (2021). "Covid-19 Lockdown Cost/Benefits: A Critical Assessment of the Literature," in

Lockdowns and social-distancing measures inflict unemployment, business collapse, education neglect, health neglect and loneliness. The virus does not do these things. Government directives do these things.

Summing the costs

Table 1.1 below summarises the costs of lockdowns in **WELLBYs per month** for Australia, with data sourced from the ensuing chapters of this report.

Category	Disrupted area	Costs in original units on average per month for 2020, 2021	Costs in WELLBYs on average per month for 2020, 2021	Costs beyond 2021
Lost GDP and increased expenditure	Economic loss	$8.045 billion per month	482,700 WELLBYs per month	
Lost well-being	Lost well-being (life satisfaction)	Drop in life satisfaction of 0.2 on a 0-10 scale on average per year of stop-start lockdowns	428,334 WELLBYs per month	
	Non-COVID excess deaths in 2020 and 2021	7,940 additional non-COVID deaths from lockdowns in the first two years of the pandemic	9,937 WELLBYs per month	
Future costs	Reduction in the general lifespan of all Australians	Loss of one week of life for the average Australian		59,304 WELLBYs per year for the next 50 years
	Lost future productivity of children born during lockdowns	Lifetime earnings of 600,000 children born during 2020 and 2021 drops by $18 billion (or $30,000 per child) over a 35-year working life due to reduced IQ; a total WELLBY loss of 1,080,000 WELLBYs		30,857 WELLBYs per year starting in 20 years and continuing for the ensuing 35 years

International Journal of the Economics of Business, DOI: 10.1080/13571516.2021.1976051, https://www.tandfonline.com/doi/abs/10.1080/13571516.2021.1976051).

	Lost future productivity of children of school age during lockdowns	$465 million in lost lifetime earnings of schoolchildren (27,900 WELLBYs over 35 years of working life)		797 WELLBYs per year (27900/35) starting in 10 years and continuing for the ensuing 35 years

Table 1.1: Summary of the estimated short-term and longer-term costs of Australia's lockdowns and border closures

The first three rows, showing estimates of costs paid during the lockdown period, average out to 920,971 WELLBYs per month, or 920,971 x 24 = **22.10 million WELLBYs in all over two years.**

The next three rows present the tally of future costs of the lockdowns implemented in 2020 and 2021 and are discounted in order to be comparable with other lockdown costs which are expressed in "2021 well-being currency." The present value of these future costs at a 5% yearly discount rate is **1.31 million WELLBYs.**

The sum of these two cost estimates, **23.41 million WELLBYs,** is the total estimated cost of lockdowns in 2021 well-being currency.

The spreadsheet containing the net present value calculations underpinning these figures is available on the internet for public perusal.[31]

1.2.4 *Cost-benefit ratio*

Choosing conservatively to exclude or under-estimate many costs, and to make generous estimates of benefits, I estimate the maximum benefits from Australia's lockdown policies to be **343,800** WELLBYs, and the minimum costs from lockdowns to be **23.41 million WELLBYs.**

This indicates that **the costs of Australia's COVID lockdowns have been at least 68 times greater than the benefits they delivered.** Because I make assumptions in this CBA that are extremely favourable to the government's choice to pursue a lockdown strat-

---

[31] http://sanjeev.sabhlokcity.com/Misc/Final-cost-table-CBA.xlsx

egy, the true ratio of costs to benefits of the Australian COVID lockdowns is likely to be greater than this.

1.3 Opportunity costs: Deaths that could have been avoided with dollars spent on COVID

Another way to evaluate the effectiveness of policies to minimise harm from COVID starts with the following question: what is the opportunity cost of the dollars we have spent on our COVID response?

According to the Australian Institute of Health and Welfare:

> Potentially avoidable deaths are deaths among people younger than 75 that are potentially avoidable within the present health care system. They include deaths from conditions that are potentially preventable through individualised care and/or treatable through existing primary or hospital care. In 2019, there were 28,000 potentially avoidable deaths: half (48%) of all deaths for people aged less than 75. Of these deaths, 64% were male and 36% were female.[32]

One could estimate quite easily how many lives could have been saved if the hundreds of billions of dollars spent by the government on lockdowns, and policies associated with the disruption they caused, had instead been spent on other health priorities. Such an exercise leads to the conclusion that if hundreds of billions of dollars had been invested in non-COVID-related health care during 2020 and 2021, instead of being used to pursue lockdowns and cushion their fallout, Australia could have avoided tens of thousands of (non-COVID) deaths. Spending some of this money on research into early treatment and/or prophylaxis of those infected with or at serious risk from COVID, respectively, could have prevented some COVID deaths.[33] Estimating how many lives could have been saved by pur-

---

[32] Australian Institute of Health and Welfare (2021). "Deaths in Australia - Web report," last updated: 25 Jun 2021, https://bit.ly/3wzA2tG.

[33] Early treatments have been identified by various experts since 2020. For example (a) https://bit.ly/3NvfDLT: "COVID-19 early treatment: real-time analysis of 1,811 studies," in which the authors note: "Denying efficacy increases mortality, morbidity, and collateral damage"; (b) Alexander, P.E. (2022): "Early Outpatient Treatment for COVID-19: The Evidence," Brownstone Institute, 22 January 2022, https://archive.ph/B6VlY. Also see c19early.com.

suing a "best-practice" prophylaxis and treatment regime in place of lockdowns would be of high social value but is beyond the scope of this report.

1.4 Limitations of this study

Like any cost-benefit analysis, this document is not definitive. I expect many of the costs imposed by lockdowns, particularly through the unintended consequences of these policies, to become clearer and more measurable over time. Individual line items will need to be updated, but more broadly, future researchers bear the responsibility to attempt the difficult task of valuing the intangible costs of the Australian lockdowns to Australians' stance towards their government and society. Such costs arise from the loss of individual liberty, the fracture of communities, and the abandonment of principles of good governance and public health stewardship as our governments became propagandists. I hope that future research will deliver estimates of the cost of the marginal changes to trust and belief in government, in our institutions (including public health), and in one another, that lockdowns have wrought.

While the list and magnitude of costs is expected to expand with time, few new benefits of lockdowns are likely to emerge. This is because the plausible benefits of lockdowns, and those on the basis of which they were originally defended, are mainly those occurring in the short run (i.e., during the lockdowns themselves). Consequently, I do not expect my conclusion that net damage was done to Australia by lockdowns to be reversed by future information. I suspect, instead, that the adverse assessment of lockdowns illustrated in this CBA is likely to worsen. I have characterised the COVID lockdowns of this era as a mass sacrificial event,[34] and I sadly expect future data and research merely to re-confirm this assessment.

---

[34] Patrick, Aaron (2021). "COVID-19 lockdowns a 'mass sacrificial event,'" in *Financial Review*, 16 July 2021. https://archive.ph/mD38o.

PART 1

BACKGROUND DISCUSSION

2. Public policy principles in Australia

The need for good policy processes is particularly acute when facing a public health crisis. Australia has long incorporated some of the world's best principles in its public policy development.

2.1 Basic principles of public policy development

The 2019 edition of the *Victorian Guide to Regulation* (VGR) notes that "It is not possible for governments to provide a completely 'risk free' society, or to prevent every possible event that might cause harm." Further: "the direct and indirect costs imposed by regulatory approaches may not be ... immediately obvious. Risk regulation that is poorly targeted or costly will divert resources from other priorities."[35]

The VGR identifies seven best-practice principles to guide regulation, as shown in the box below.

Principles for regulation in Victoria

The Government is committed to the following best practice regulatory principles to guide the design, implementation and review of all regulatory proposals and changes to existing regulations in Victoria.

The Government requires regulations to be:

- effective in addressing the underlying causes of harm
- cost effective
- proportionate to the harm or risk to the community
- flexible to accommodate changes in technology, markets, risks and community views
- consistent with the Government's priorities to enhance Victoria's liveability and growth in productivity and enmployment
- consistent across Government to avoid unnecessary overlap and duplication
- clear and easily understood by business and the community

---

[35] Commissioner for Better Regulation (2016). *Victorian Guide to Regulation*, https://bit.ly/3PAuF5a.

I discuss a few of these and related policy design principles below, and then evaluate briefly whether the policy process that led to lockdowns conformed to these principles.

2.1.1 *The need to understand the nature and causes of harm*

Policy analysis begins with a thorough understanding of the harm being allegedly addressed by the policy. The greater the clarity we develop about the harm we are addressing, the greater the prospect of identifying effective options to address it. In the case of COVID, this means understanding who is at risk and how this risk can plausibly be mitigated.

2.1.2 *Proportionality as a basic hurdle for public policy options*

In order to stay under consideration, policy options must pass a number of basic hurdles, the most essential being that of proportionality. Viable options for a policy response must neither be excessive nor insufficient.

This principle is embedded in legislation. Section 9 of Victoria's *Public Health and Wellbeing Act 2008* states: "decisions made and actions taken in the administration of this Act should be proportionate to the public health risk sought to be prevented, minimised or controlled; and should not be made or taken in an arbitrary manner."

Likewise, the 10 March 2020 Victorian pandemic plan included this principle of proportionality: to "ensure a proportionate and equitable response." The plan stated that all actions should be "flexible and proportionate." Guidance on proportionality is widely available, such as in the *User Guide to the Australian Government Guide to Regulatory Impact Analysis.*[36]

2.1.3 *Cost effectiveness of options*

Of the proportionate and hence shortlisted options available for addressing the risk of harm from a given threat, a competent govern-

---

[36] The Office of Best Practice Regulation, Department of Premier and Cabinet, Australian Government (2021). *User Guide to the Australian Government Guide to Regulatory Impact Analysis*, https://archive.ph/I2HUX.

ment identifies the most cost effective. Cost effectiveness considers not only the financial costs of a policy option, but all human (including health) costs of that option, and shows the total cost of each unit of benefit produced by the policy.

A CBA assesses all expected costs and benefits of all shortlisted options, with assumptions clearly articulated. In the case of an unexpected emergency, a short-form CBA can be undertaken and continually updated as new information becomes available and uncertainty is resolved. The involvement of economists is important to the CBA process, since economists are trained to identify and assess the social value (positive or negative) of a policy, including its less visible and often unintended consequences.

The guiding principle of a CBA is conceptually similar to the commonly expressed goal of pursuing the "greater good." If a policy option is expected to produce a positive net benefit to society (i.e., social benefits minus social costs), then the "greater good" will likely be achieved by it. The preferred option, in standard practice, would be the most cost-effective of all shortlisted options that would achieve the "greater good."

2.1.4 Dealing with uncertainty

In general, economists use the best data available at a point in time to generate estimates of the benefits and harms of a policy. In many cases, uncertainties remain, which can be gauged.

Uncertainties at the early stage of the COVID pandemic could have been modelled using probabilistic assessments of different scenarios, which in turn could have been updated regularly based on evolving empirical evidence.

2.2 Did Australian governments adhere to the above principles of good policy making?

The scientific consensus prior to March 2020, encapsulated in approved pandemic plans, was that lockdowns could at best only delay the inevitable, and at huge cost. Thus, it would have been seen as reckless to recommend lockdowns – which directly cause harms – on whole populations, even if lockdowns were effective in saving lives, if whole populations are not at risk of harm from COVID.

Before implementation, the COVID lockdown policy option should have been defended not only on the basis of delivering favourable COVID outcomes, but as having comparatively low human costs per unit of expected benefit (i.e., high cost-effectiveness). The human costs considered in this assessment should have included both immediate and future costs, recognising that every policy represents a trade-off of costs for benefits.

A process built on proportionality is embedded into Australia's laws,[37] but ordinary journalists have questioned whether lockdowns passed the test of proportionality, such as on 27 October 2020 when the editorial board of *The Australian* wrote that "the disproportionate financial and human costs of lockdown and poorly thought-through border closures are becoming more obvious by the day."[38]

Australian Ministers and senior officials (such as Queensland's Police Commissioner[39]) have justified their actions during the pandemic by claiming that these actions advance the "greater good." Yet the subjective assessments of officials are not adequate assurance that their policies are achieving the "greater good." Only a rigorous and transparent CBA can support the claim that the "greater good" is being served.

To my knowledge, no Australian government has yet released a

---

[37] Illustratively, Section 9 of Victoria's *Public Health and Wellbeing Act 2008* (https://bit.ly/3luYbv9) states that "decisions made and actions taken in the administration of this Act should be proportionate to the public health risk sought to be prevented, minimised or controlled; and should not be made or taken in an arbitrary manner." Article 12 of the Siracusa Principles on the Limitation and Derogation Provisions in the International Covenant on Civil and Political Rights (https://archive.ph/KfzMz), to which Australia is a signatory, places the justificatory burden of rights limitations on the state imposing those limitations.

[38] *The Australian* – Editorial (2020). "Open borders to rekindle the vitality of Federation," 16 October 2020, https://bit.ly/38floxo.

[39] Queensland Police Commissioner Katarina Carrol in a 9 News Australia news report on YouTube, 29 September 2021, http://youtu.be/T3ZB3o2wvUE.

CBA justifying its COVID policies, including lockdowns. The Australian people still await an explanation of why Australian governments considered lockdowns an appropriate policy response to COVID-19. This failure undermines the standard CBA-based policy process of Australia and sets an alarming precedent for the management of future pandemics.

Rather than defending lockdowns using a rigorous CBA, governments in Australia and elsewhere focused solely on COVID benefits and ignored any systematic consideration of costs. Very belatedly, on 12 May 2022, a member of the Scientific Advisory Group for Emergencies ("SAGE") in the UK admitted to this policy design failure:

> Professor John Edmunds said the models were only supposed to be 'one component' of decision-making but were leaned on too much by ministers. He accepted the models failed to account for the economic harm and the knock-on health effects that lockdowns caused. Professor Edmunds admitted that these harms 'in principle' could have been factored into models 'but in practice they were not'.[40]

2.2.1 *Calls for COVID policy that delivers net human benefit*

I have long called for a CBA of Australia's pandemic policies. In my testimony at the August 2020 meeting of Victoria's PAEC I made clear that the burden of proof to provide such analysis is on the government's shoulders. It is not up to me or others questioning the imposition of the government's radical measures to prove that such measures are not a good idea. It is the government's responsibility to defend its radical measures on the basis that they in fact promote human welfare. Interventions of an unprecedented scale like lockdowns are uncharted territory, meaning that stronger justification for them than for a "normal" policy would have been expected. Accountability to the people who have put policy makers in power, and on whom those lockdowns were imposed, means transparently estimating the

---

[40] *Daily Mail.* "SAGE models were too 'scary' and held too much weight... says lockdown architect behind them! No10 Covid expert admits death forecasts were 'eye watering' and should have considered economy," 12 May 2022, https://archive.ph/7Viff.

human welfare costs of lockdowns as well as their benefits. As part of this process of demonstrating accountability, governments should have at least nodded to the ethical and human rights challenges posed by the extreme policy of lockdowns, even if such challenges are not formally quantified as part of the CBA.

On 13 August 2020 the philosopher Peter Singer, a Laureate Professor at the Centre for Applied Philosophy and Public Ethics at the University of Melbourne, is reported to have expressed surprise that governments had taken such strong actions without presenting cost benefit analyses.[41]

Peter Singer also remarked on the need to recognise the number of years of life lost, not just the number of deaths: "That it's less tragic for a 90-year-old to die than a 30-year-old seems clear to me." Singer advised the outright rejection of the approach of health professionals like Devi Sridhar who suggest valuing all lives equally,[42] noting that it is "totally reasonable" for governments to assign a value to human life for the purposes of allocating public spending. "Otherwise you get irrational decisions where the department of road safety spends $8m to save a life whereas you could save $4m [sic: meaning "spend $4m to save a life"] in another [area]."

Consistent with the standard Australian health policy-making process, The University of Melbourne's Vice-Chancellor Duncan Maskell said on 19 September 2020 that "decision-makers must consider the role of quality-adjusted life year (QALY), a unit of measurement used by economists to predict and assess the impact of health policies. In simple terms, it assumes that a life near its end, whether because of disease or advanced age, is empirically different to a healthy life closer to its beginning."[43] This principle is embedded into the analysis presented in this document.

---

[41] Creighton, Adam (2020), "Lockdowns could eventually be seen as an over-reaction, says philosopher Peter Singer," in *The Australian*, 13 August 2020, https://bit.ly/337i6rK.
[42] Tweet dated 5 April 2020 by Devi Sridhar, https://bit.ly/3yLSsJk.
[43] Le Grand, Chip (2020), "Melbourne Uni chief says Victoria must address difficult ethical questions," in *The Sydney Morning Herald*, 19 September 2020, https://bit.ly/38LQuhs.

3. Nature and magnitude of the COVID disease

To create a proportionate response to a problem, we need an accurate gauge of its nature and magnitude. This chapter presents an analysis of the nature and magnitude of COVID-19 as a threat to human life and health.

3.1 Nature of the COVID disease

Two features of COVID-19 have been known since at least February 2020: (a) its mortality risks are skewed towards the elderly; and (b) within age groups, COVID adversely affects mainly those with multiple co-morbidities.[44]

3.1.1 *COVID risks are skewed towards the elderly*

The age-dependent risk profile of COVID has not changed over the past two years. It remains largely a non-event in healthy children but carries a serious risk of death for the elderly, particularly in the presence of comorbidities.

Figure 3.1, taken from the Department of Health's website on 27 May 2022, re-confirms COVID's age-based risk profile. The very young are at extremely low risk of death. Males are more vulnerable at all ages except for the very elderly, which is likely explained by the higher life expectancy of females. These realities are apparent in mortality statistics released by the Australian Bureau of Statistics.[45]

---

[44] *China CDC Weekly* (2020). "Vital Surveillances: The Epidemiological Characteristics of an Outbreak of 2019 Novel Coronavirus Diseases (COVID-19) – China, 2020," 2(8): 113-122, https://bit.ly/3cSQCNY, 17 February 2020. This paper reports that "The ≥80 age group had the highest case fatality rate of all age groups at 14.8%."

[45] Australian Bureau of Statistics (2022). COVID-19 Mortality in Australia: Deaths registered until 31 March 2022, https://bit.ly/38nx2Hx.

Source: NINDSS data 15/8/2022

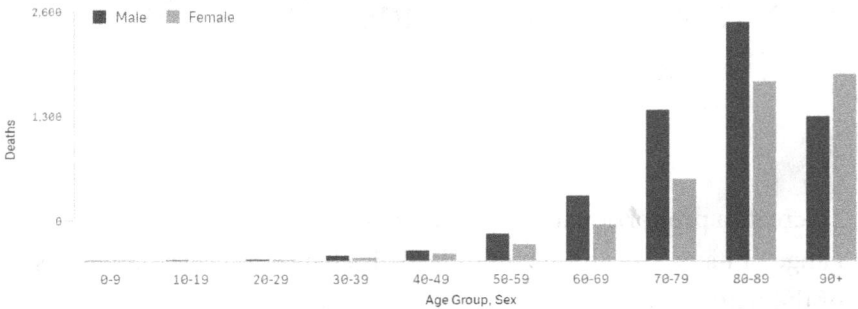

Figure 3.1: The risk profile of COVID[46]

While Australia's sample size of COVID deaths is relatively small, larger datasets from other nations show a similar pattern (e.g., in the USA[47]).

3.1.2 *The role of co-morbidities*

Within each age group, COVID is a lethal threat mainly to those with multiple co-morbidities. This was known early: on 18 March 2020 it was reported that "More than 99% of Italy's coronavirus fatalities were people who suffered from previous medical conditions, according to a study by the country's national health authority."[48] Further:

> A subsample of 355 patients with COVID-19 who died in Italy underwent detailed chart review. Among these patients, the mean age was 79.5 years (SD, 8.1) and 106 (30.0%) were women. In this sample, 117 patients (30%) had ischemic heart disease, 126 (35.5%) had diabetes, 72 (20.3%) had active cancer, 87 (24.5%) had atrial fibrillation, 24 (6.8%) had dementia, and 34 (9.6%) had a history of stroke. The mean number of preexisting diseases was 2.7 (SD, 1.6). Overall, only 3 patients (0.8%) had no diseases, 89 (25.1%) had a

---

[46] Department of Health, Australian Government (2022). Coronavirus (COVID-19) case numbers and statistics, https://bit.ly/3PNtBuA.

[47] Centres for Disease Control and Prevention. COVID-19 Mortality Overview. https://bit.ly/3wAYf2O.

[48] Bloomberg (2020). "99% of Those Who Died From Virus Had Other Illness, Italy Says," 18 March 2020, https://bit.ly/3PElPTJ.

single disease, 91 (25.6%) had 2 diseases, and 172 (48.5%) had 3 or more underlying diseases. The presence of these comorbidities might have increased the risk of mortality in-dependent of COVID-19 infection.[49]

On 8 June 2020 it was reported that: "The number and severity of these co-[morbidities] has been a major factor influencing the out-come; this was particularly evident where the virus diffused into old pension homes."[50]

This strong association with co-morbidities is evident not only for the risk of death, but for the risk of serious outcomes. The United States CDC analysed nearly half a million hospitalisations of patients with COVID and found that nearly two-thirds of the hospitalised had over six co-morbidities (Figure 3.2).

Table 1. Characteristics of Adults Hospitalized With COVID-19 in Premier Healthcare Database Special COVID-19 Release (PHD-SR), March 2020–March 2021

Characteristic[a]	All Hospitalized Patients in PHD-SR, No. (%)	Hospitalized Patients With COVID-19, No. (%)			
		Full Sample	ICU[b] admission	IMV[b]	Died[b]
Total	4,899,447 (100.0)	540,667 (100.0)	249,522 (100.0)	76,680 (100.0)	80,174 (100.0)
No. of conditions					
≥1[c]	4,438,183 (90.6)	513,292 (94.9)	242,372 (97.1)	75,514 (98.5)	79,434 (99.1)
0	461,264 (9.4)	27,375 (5.1)	7,150 (2.9)	1,166 (1.5)	740 (0.9)
1	402,499 (8.2)	39,776 (7.4)	14,272 (5.7)	2,785 (3.6)	2,087 (2.6)
2–5	1,796,770 (36.7)	212,429 (39.3)	94,405 (37.8)	27,405 (35.7)	25,893 (32.3)
6–10	1,565,845 (32.0)	167,706 (31.0)	84,745 (34.0)	28,774 (37.5)	31,310 (39.1)
>10	673,069 (13.7)	93,381 (17.3)	48,950 (19.6)	16,550 (21.6)	20,144 (25.1)

Figure 3.2: 64.2% of those hospitalised with COVID had more than six co-morbidities.[51]

This suggests that healthy individuals have far less to fear from CO-VID than unhealthy ones. An appropriate policy response to COVID would logically have taken this reality into account. Sanjeev Sabhlok suggested such a proportionate policy response on 6 March 2020,[52]

---

[49] Onder, et al (2020). "Case-Fatality Rate and Characteristics of Patients Dying in Relation to COVID-19 in Italy," in *Jama Network*, 23 March 2020, https://jamanetwork.com/journals/jama/fullarticle/2763667.

[50] Chen, Jun et al (2020). "COVID-19 infection: the China and Italy perspectives," in *Cell Death & Disease*, 11, Article 438 (2020). https://www.nature.com/articles/s41419-020-2603-0.

[51] Kompaniyets L., et al (2021). "Underlying Medical Conditions and Severe Illness Among 540,667 Adults Hospitalized With COVID-19, March 2020–March 2021," in *Preventing Chronic Disease*, 2021;18:210123. DOI: https://doi.org/10.5888/pcd18.210123.

[52] Sabhlok, Sanjeev (2020). "Age-based risk management of coronavirus," in *The Times of India* blog, 6 March 2020, https://bit.ly/3PtNV42.

I opined similarly on national radio later that month,[53] and Victoria's 10 March 2020 pandemic plan also advised taking such an approach, with its principles "[f]ocused on protecting vulnerable Victorians, including with underlying health conditions, compromised immune systems, the elderly, Aboriginal and Torres Strait Islanders, and those from culturally and linguistically diverse communities."[54] This was also the approach followed by Sweden, with *Science* reporting on 6 October 2020 that "[Anders] Tegnell has said repeatedly that the Swedish strategy takes a holistic view of public health, aiming to balance the risk of the virus with the damage from countermeasures like closed schools. The goal was to protect the elderly and other high-risk groups while slowing viral spread enough to avoid hospitals being overwhelmed." In October 2020, the authors of the Great Barrington Declaration[55] called this the "focussed protection" approach.

3.1.3 *Mortality risk correlates inversely with vitamin D3 status*

While pre-COVID literature showed that vitamin D plays a role in fighting respiratory viruses like the flu,[56] over the past two years we have learned that vitamin D sufficiency also correlates with better COVID outcomes. The role of vitamin D sufficiency has policy implications because dietary supplementation and/or sun exposure, which produces vitamin D, can be made into recommendations for the community.

The pre-2020 science literature showed that vitamin D strengthens innate immunity to respiratory viruses, while moderating potentially excessive responsivity of the adaptive immune system, thus reducing cytokine storms which cause harm. On the basis of

[53] Australian Broadcasting Company, Radio National (2020). "As the coronavirus marches on, can wartime measures save us from a depression?" Interview with Gigi Foster and others, 26 March 2020, https://archive.ph/uU0BE.
[54] Mikakos, Jenny (MP) (2020). *COVID-19 Pandemic plan for the Victorian Health Sector*, Version 1.0, 10 March 2020, https://bit.ly/3wJEnti.
[55] Great Barrington Declaration (2020), 4 October 2020, https://gbdeclaration.org/.
[56] E.g., *The Harvard Gazette* (2017). "Study confirms vitamin D protects against colds and flu," https://bit.ly/3ak0P4t.

this, many scientists at the commencement of the pandemic advocated higher intake of vitamin D as a plausible, low-cost way to reduce COVID deaths.[57] Dr David Grimes of the UK informed Sanjeev Sabhlok in April 2022 that he worked with the British Association of Physicians of Indian Origin in early 2020 to send a circular to its members to increase vitamin D intake, which he then said stopped COVID deaths among dark-skinned doctors in the UK.[58]

Evidence suggesting a link between vitamin D insufficiency and the risk of dying from COVID includes:

- On 1 October 2020, an article in the *Daily Mail* reported that "dozens" of studies showed a strong protective effect from COVID disease of vitamin D sufficiency.[59]

- On 17 June 2021, a report about an Israeli study stated that "1 in 4 covid patients hospitalized while vitamin D deficient die."[60]

- On 14 October 2021, a peer reviewed paper in *Nutrients*[61] noted that "low D3 is a predictor rather than just a side effect of the infection. Despite ongoing vaccinations, we recommend raising serum 25(OH)D levels to above 50 ng/mL to prevent or mitigate

---

[57] For example, see the April 2020 paper by Grant, William B. et al, "Evidence that Vitamin D Supplementation Could Reduce Risk of Influenza and COVID-19 Infections and Deaths," in *Nutrients* vol. 12(4):988, doi:10.3390/nu12040988 and an April 2020 report by Trinity College Dublin: "Vitamin D could help fight off Covid-19 – new TILDA research" (https://bit.ly/3LzPKJK). Since then, the role of vitamin D has been more clearly established – see for example, "Patients with vitamin D deficiency (<20 ng/mL) were 14 times more likely to have severe or critical disease than patients with 25(OH)D ≥40 ng/mL" (https://bit.ly/3NrRW7b).

[58] Sabhlokcity. "Claim that Vitamin D brought to a halt in the death of Indian doctors in the UK – Dr David Grimes," 7 April 2022, https://bit.ly/3NAOPtO.

[59] Boyd, Connor (2020). "Since the Covid-19 epidemic started multiple studies have repeatedly shown a link to Vitamin D deficiency yet when Matt Hancock was asked about it he WRONGLY said a British study had found the opposite. Is he ignorant or incompetent?" in *Daily Mail Online,* 1 October 2020, https://bit.ly/3Pu8ihH.

[60] Jeffay, Nathan (2021), "1 in 4 COVID patients hospitalized while vitamin D deficient die – Israeli study," in *The Times of Israel*, 12 June 2021, https://archive.ph/rDpYI.

[61] Borsche, Lorenz, Bernd Glauner, and Julian von Mendel (2021). "COVID-19 Mortality Risk Correlates Inversely with Vitamin D3 Status, and a Mortality Rate Close to Zero Could Theoretically Be Achieved at 50 ng/mL 25(OH)D3: Results of a Systematic Review and Meta-Analysis," in *Nutrients* 13, no. 10: 3596, https://doi.org/10.3390/nu13103596.

new outbreaks due to escape mutations or decreasing antibody activity."

The potential downsides of vitamin D intake – such as massive overdosing resulting in toxicity, or sunburn – are likely manageable enough that a favourable risk-benefit case could be made. Vitamin D supplements are reasonably cheap and sun exposure is free. If the role of vitamin D in protecting against severe COVID outcomes was even suspected to be positive, the Australian government should have encouraged greater exposure of people to the sun and/or advised vitamin D supplementation, particularly for vulnerable groups.[62]

3.1.4 *Other risk factors*

Many other likely risk factors for COVID have been identified over the past two years, such as previous exposure to coronaviruses (due to cross-reactivity of the immune response[63]) reducing severity, and density of housing (e.g., dense, multi-story housing) likely to increase the spread.[64]

---

[62] Sabhlok, Sanjeev (2020). "The effect of innate immunity, cross-reactivity, trained immunity and vitamin D on Covid-19," in *The Times of India* blog, 24 May 2020, https://bit.ly/3wHZrjJ.

[63] In an article in *ScienceMag* on 15 May 2020 entitled, "Good News on the Human Immune Response to the Coronavirus," Derek Lowe noted that cross-reactivity was "a big factor in making the H1N1 flu epidemic less severe than had been initially feared – the population already had more of an immunological head start than thought." It would be reasonable to expect something similar to be true for the coronavirus we call COVID. Dr Sunetra Gupta, professor of theoretical epidemiology at Oxford University, suggested in an interview on *UnHerd* on 21 May 2020 that humanity has very strong innate and cross-reactivity to COVID. A 14 May 2020 paper entitled, "Targets of T cell responses to SARS-CoV-2 coronavirus in humans with COVID-19 disease and unexposed individuals" noted that "we detected SARS-CoV-2–reactive CD4+ T cells in ~ 40-60% of unexposed individuals, suggesting cross-reactive T cell recognition between circulating 'common cold' coronaviruses and SARS-CoV-2" (https://pubmed.ncbi.nlm.nih.gov/32473127/). A 23 July 2020 paper entitled "Pre-existing and de novo humoral immunity to SARS-CoV-2 in humans" provides further evidence for cross-reactivity through which protection from COVID (via SARS-CoV-2 neutralising antibodies) is provided by the natural immune system as a result of prior exposure to other things, such as common-cold coronaviruses, particularly in children.

[64] Examples of the rapid spread of COVID in 2020 within a dense environment include the Diamond Princess cruise ship experience (https://www.nature.com/articles/d41586-020-00885-w) and the case of high-rise buildings in Hong Kong. The aerosol mechanism for rapid transmission in high-rise buildings, which could not manifest in more spread-out areas such as single-home

Summarising what we know as of May 2022, the risk of an adverse event from COVID infection is particularly high for those over 80 and/or those with co-morbidities such as diabetes and obesity, and the virus is likely to cause more damage in the presence of vitamin D insufficiency, low prior coronavirus exposure, and lifestyle factors that promote transmission to the vulnerable and/or reduce individual immune strength. The risk posed by COVID-19 infection is very low for healthy young people and approaches zero in children. Finally, not being treated for COVID infection is itself a major risk factor for developing more serious disease, particularly in the vulnerable.[65]

3.2   Magnitude of the COVID pandemic

3.2.1 *The opinion of experts and official pandemic plans*

As with the risk profile of COVID across individuals, the overall magnitude of the threat it posed was reasonably well understood by early 2020. Victoria's pandemic plan of 10 March 2020 confirmed that "COVID-19 is assessed as being of moderate clinical severity."[66] This plan did not limit its guidance only to handling a pandemic of moderate severity. It stated that "we are preparing so that we are ready to respond if a larger, or more severe outbreak occurs." No "larger" or "more severe" outbreaks than what would be categorised as "moderate severity" ever occurred anywhere in Australia in 2020 or 2021.[67]

residential zones in suburban and regional Australia, is elaborated upon in a January 2022 paper available at https://pubmed.ncbi.nlm.nih.gov/34396958/.

[65] For a review of what was known about the efficacy of early treatment options at the start of 2022, see Alexander, P.E. (2022). "Early Outpatient Treatment for COVID-19: The Evidence," Brownstone Institute, 22 January 2022, https://archive.ph/B6VlY.

[66] The Victorian Government's "COVID-19 Pandemic Plan for the Victorian Health Sector" (10 March 2020) is no longer available from the Victorian Government's original website (https://bit.ly/3G61X7C), but a copy of the plan is available at https://bit.ly/3wJEnti.

[67] Clinical severity criteria are not elaborated upon in the Victorian pandemic plan, but the Australian plan at https://bit.ly/3LzzGHN notes that "[t]he clinical severity of the disease will affect the number of people that present to primary care, and who need to be hospitalised." While there were some reports of a few developing countries being temporarily overwhelmed during a COVID peak, it was rare for the reasonably well-

Even as modelers were delivering very high estimates of the threat,[68] with the media joining in, experts like John Ioannidis were recommending caution and suggesting the virus might not be as big a problem as was being claimed. On 17 March 2020, he wrote:

> The current coronavirus disease, Covid-19, has been called a once-in-a-century pandemic. But it may also be a once-in-a-century evidence fiasco.... [R]easonable estimates for the case fatality ratio in the general U.S. population vary from 0.05% to 1%" ... we don't know how long social distancing measures and lockdowns can be maintained without major consequences to the economy, society, and mental health. If we decide to jump off the cliff, we need some data to inform us about the rationale of such an action and the chances of landing somewhere safe.[69]

By contrast, the Prime Minister of Australia claimed on 18 March 2020 that, "This is a once-in-a-hundred-year type event. We haven't seen this sort of thing in Australia since the end of the First World War."[70] Such rhetoric has been the norm in Australia during the pandemic, with extreme claims of this kind repeated by many people in positions of power. As another example, Chief Health Officer of Victoria, Brett Sutton, claimed on 12 July 2020 that we were facing the "greatest public health challenge since the Spanish flu."[71]

established health systems of developed Western nations to come under substantial stress in 2020. Sweden experienced a minor overload in some ICUs during the second peak in December 2020-January 2021 and transferred excess patients to nearby ICUs which had capacity. In the US it was not so much that hospitals were overwhelmed, but that they were forcibly closed off to most work by government edict (Tucker, Jeffrey A. (2021). "Why Did Healthcare Spending Decline 8.6% During a Pandemic?" Brownstone Institute, 17 June 2021, https://archive.ph/2HLOA).

[68] It appears that after being empirically driven in early March 2020, Victoria's policy choices regressed to using model-based simulations that grossly over-stated the severity of the pandemic ("Theoretical modelling to inform Victoria's response to coronavirus (COVID-19)," https://bit.ly/3wzvcMV).

[69] Ioannidis, John P.A. (2020). "A fiasco in the making? As the coronavirus pandemic takes hold, we are making decisions without reliable data," in *STAT News*, 17 March 2020, https://bit.ly/3wyu4ta.

[70] Prime Minister of Australia (2020). Transcript of Press Conference – Australian Parliament House ACT, 18 March 2020. https://bit.ly/3LzAbSb.

[71] Carey, Adam, and Webb, Carolyn (2020). "Remote-learning move not enough to quell teachers' virus fears," in *The Age*, 12 July 2020, https://archive.ph/IIVw3.

3.2.2 *COVID is not in the league of the Spanish flu*

COVID was known early on not to be comparable to the Spanish flu. According to the CDC's website, there were "at least" 50 million global deaths in 1918-1919 from the Spanish flu when the world's population was 1.8 billion.[72] The current world population is 7.9 billion. Therefore, around 219 million people would need to die from COVID in order to credibly claim that the COVID pandemic is in the league of the Spanish flu, simply in terms of death counts alone. Even then, a comparison would be misguided, because the two viruses have starkly different risk profiles by age: Spanish flu frequently killed healthy young people, whereas COVID mainly kills the old and sick, and this was known in March 2020.

The 6.3 million deaths with COVID being reported by Worldometer as at 27 May 2022 represent more than 30 times fewer deaths than 219 million. There is no comparison between the two pandemics: not in terms of body counts, and not in terms of risk profiles by age. Figure 1.1 depicts the relative magnitude of four pandemics of the past hundred years.[73]

Even if we accept the unlikely proposition that all reported CO-VID deaths were caused by COVID (a dubious claim, as illustrated by the fact that in 2020, excess deaths in Sweden totalled less than a third of reported COVID deaths[74]), the COVID pandemic is at worst in the range of the Asian flu of 1957, for which the world did not shut down. A review in Chapter 4 of this report of the pre-2020 scientific consensus about how to respond to pandemics indicates

---

[72] Centers for Disease Control and Prevention, "1918 Pandemic (H1N1 virus)" – website as at 20 May 2022, https://bit.ly/3Lvztp2.

[73] *Source* – data and chart: https://bit.ly/3ut40LA.

[74] "Excess mortality due to Covid-19? A comparison of total mortality in 2020 with total mortality in 2016 to 2019 in Germany, Sweden and Spain," by Bernd Kowall et al in *PLoS ONE*, https://journals.plos.org/plosone/article?id=10.1371/journal.pone.0255540, found that in 2020 Sweden experienced excess mortality of 3%, or around 3,000 extra deaths, consistent with the estimate of Nobel laureate Michael Levitt of 3%, available at https://bit.ly/38BA0sk. 10,000 deaths were reported in Sweden in 2020 as COVID deaths.

that even if the COVID pandemic had been as severe a threat as the Spanish flu, lockdowns would not have been justified. If ever used, they should only have been implemented on as limited a scale as possible and on the basis of a robust analysis concluding that their known harms would be outweighed by their plausible benefits.

3.2.3 *Contextualising the magnitude of the problem*

Another way to contextualise the magnitude of the pandemic is offered below.

a) 98.975% of the world's population survived the year 2020. Of the 7800-odd million people in the world at the beginning of 2020, 2 million reportedly died with/from COVID, representing 0.025% of the global population.

b) During the same year, 2020, the global population grew by approximately 80 million.

These numbers illustrate that the extreme actions of governments worldwide (excluding a small number of regions, such as Sweden) could not have been the result of reasoned risk assessment. Professor John Lee writes on the biases involved:

> Many people have the impression of this epidemic that they have because of the initial framing. The initial framing was one of panic. The authorities were panicked. Many professionals were panicked by the idea of a very serious virulent disease coming out of China. We haven't really had a revision of it. The authorities, in my opinion, have painted themselves into a corner by their responses to covid and they really have been forced to stick to the narrative that they invented to start with.
>
> There's a thing called ascertainment bias. At the beginning of an epidemic you identify the most serious cases first because they're the ones who turn up in hospitals but they are at the far end of the spectrum in terms of severity. So, what normally happens is as an epidemic progresses and more and more people catch the disease it turns out that the disease is not as severe as people thought it was going to be. And so,

the infection fatality rate falls and that's exactly what's happened with COVID.[75]

3.2.4 *Epidemiological models grossly exaggerated the likely severity of the pandemic*

In 2020, a vocal sub-group of epidemiologists produced models of viral spread that caused great confusion. Their models grossly exag-gerated potential COVID deaths. Policy makers, alarmed by these models that also alarmed the public, chose to take extreme actions purportedly to combat the "worst-case scenario," even though simi-lar modelling of viral pathogens had proven in past decades to have been wildly off-base.[76]

Commenting on the inappropriate use of models, Dr Sunetra Gupta observed on 15 September 2021 that "[w]hat we risk, as a scientific community, is the confidence people have in vaccines and mathematical modelling, if we push them beyond their limits."[77]

Figure 3.3 below, a chart prepared by Nick Hudson of the PANDA Institute in South Africa,[78] compares model projections for Sweden with actual deaths in 2020.[79] This suggests that epidemiological mod-

---

[75] Documentary *UK Unlocked*: http://youtu.be/btWfAXQ8wYg ("BRILLIANT: Dr John Lee, Prof of Pathology UK – Unlocked Documentary!").

[76] In 2005, Neil Ferguson predicted that up to 150 million people could be killed from bird flu. In the end, only 282 people died worldwide from the disease between 2003 and 2009. In 2009, a government estimate, based on Ferguson's advice, said a "reasonable worst-case scenario" was that the swine flu would lead to 65,000 British deaths. In the end, swine flu killed 457 people in the UK (Fund, John (2020). "'Profes-sor Lockdown' Modeler Resigns in Disgrace" in *National Review*, 6 May 2020, https://bit.ly/3NuW1I0). In the case of AIDS, the US Public Health Service announced (with-out documenting their source) that there would be 450,000 American cases by the end of 1993 (https://bit.ly/3PBgVH1), with 100,000 in that year alone. In fact, there were 17,325 American cases in total by the end of that year, with about 5,000 in 1993. SARS (2002-2003) was supposed to kill perhaps 'millions', based on analyses. It actually killed 744 before disappearing (Fumento, Michael (2020), "After Repeated Failures, It's Time To Permanently Dump Epidemic Models," in *Issues and Insights*, 18 April 2020, https://bit.ly/3ag6Xed).

[77] Tweet by The Great Barrington Declaration, 15 September 2021, https://bit.ly/3Pzj1r2.

[78] Hudson, Nick (2021). "Lockdowns don't save lives and Sweden is all the proof you need," in Pandemics Data & Analytics, 21 February 2021, https://bit.ly/3wKf6k1.

[79] Projections are drawn from Gardner, Jasmine M., et al (2020), "Intervention strate-gies against COVID-19 and their estimated impact on Swedish healthcare capacity"

els should not be used an input to pandemic policy-making without also setting in place a stringent empirical evaluation process.

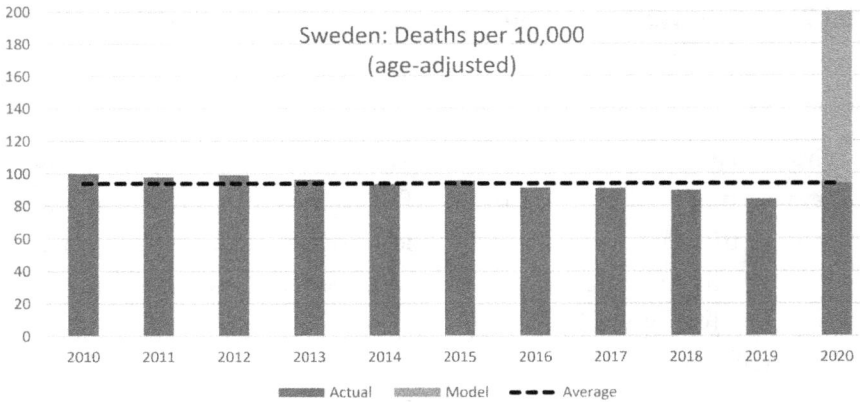

Figure 3.3: The death rate in Sweden from 2010 to 2020, including a comparison between year-2020 modelling and reality

Such over-estimation by models continued throughout the pandemic. On 20 November 2020,[80] the *Daily Mail* assessed the UK government's prediction made 20 days earlier in a 31 October 2020 press conference and found that actual deaths were lower than the predictions from any of the four models cited by the UK government to justify lockdowns. Many models predicted the duration of the second wave reasonably well, although the Imperial College London model was off by some months. However, the magnitude of all predictions was off by a wide margin, with every single model over-estimating total COVID deaths. Some estimated three to four times the number of deaths that actually occurred. More damning still, none of these models took into account deaths caused directly, now and in the future, by the proposed policy response – i.e., lockdowns.

(https://www.medrxiv.org/content/10.1101/2020.04.11.20062133v1.full.pdf), which claimed that "Our model for Sweden shows that, under conservative epidemiological parameter estimates, the current Swedish public-health strategy will result in a peak intensive-care load in May that exceeds pre-pandemic capacity by over 40-fold, with a median mortality of 96,000 (95% CI 52,000 to 183,000)."

[80] Clark, Ross (2020). "What they DON'T tell you about Covid: Fewer beds taken up than last year, deaths a fraction of the grim forecasts, 95% of fatalities had underlying causes ... and how the facts can be twisted to strike fear in our hearts," in *Daily Mail*, 20 November 2020. https://bit.ly/3sLrJbW.

The Spectator monitors the performance of models used by SAGE, the core body advising the UK government on COVID policy. The 20 November 2021 SAGE report[81] showed the dramatic exaggeration of likely hospitalisations by models in comparison with what ultimately transpired.

Inaccurate modelling was rampant not just abroad, but in Australia too. On 5 November 2021, Nine News reported that "[b]ack in September the Burnett Institute modelled that NSW would have 3,434 people in hospital with COVID and 947 in ICU by the start of November. The modelling was wildly wrong. Instead there are just 302 in hospital with COVID and 64 in ICU."[82]

In my book *The Great Covid Panic* co-written with Paul Frijters and Michael Baker,[83] we note that predictions of fatalities made during the pandemic were woefully off. The models of Neil Ferguson and his associates at Imperial College London are the poster children for this. ICL's 16 March 2020 calculations took the "advertised" case fatality rate ("CFR") of 3% and translated this into an infection fatality rate ("IFR") of 0.9%.[84] This was a fundamental blunder, as shown by the IFR of 0.096%, an order of magnitude lower, estimated by official UK sources in August 2021.[85] The ICL models still used high-end IFR rates as proxies for the estimated fatality rates of a whole exposed population as late as October 2020.[86]

When such models became dominant, the burden of proof be-

---

[81] *The Spectator* data tracker. SAGE scenarios, https://bit.ly/3LACjcr.

[82] Tweet dated 4 November 2021 by John Ruddick, https://bit.ly/3wEwEg8.

[83] https://www.thegreatcovidpanic.com/. *The Great Covid Panic: What Happened, Why, And What To Do Next*, by Paul Frijters, Gigi Foster and Michael Baker. The Brownstone Institute, 2021.

[84] Ferguson, Neil M. et al (2020). "Report 9 - Impact of non-pharmaceutical interventions (NPIs) to reduce COVID-19 mortality and healthcare demand," Imperial College London, 1-20. 10.25561/77482, 16 March 2020, https://archive.ph/rYb9C.

[85] UK Parliament, Written questions, answers and statements (2021). Coronavirus: Death, Question for Department of Health and Social Care, UIN 31381, tabled on 12 July 2021, https://bit.ly/3NrSOst.

[86] Brazeau, Nicholas F. et al (2020). "Report 34 – COVID-19 Infection Fatality Ratio Estimates from Seroprevalence," Imperial College COVID-19 Response Team1-18. 10.25561/83545, https://bit.ly/38MwLOH.

came reversed, with critics told in effect to 'prove that this published IFR does not measure the population exposure fatality rate.' That is how the scientific game came to be played in the COVID period.

Epidemiological models tend to go awry partly because they make assumptions about the pathogen that are impossible to estimate accurately. Further, the underpinning mathematics of these models are imperfect. Nobel Prize-winning scientist Michael Levitt has remarked that these models assume exponential growth, while he thinks a Gompertz curve would better capture the transmission pattern of disease outbreaks.[87] The Gompertz function starts climbing at its fastest growth rate and from there forever slows down, leading to a pattern of deaths which is relatively more consistent with actual observed "waves" than what standard models assume.[88]

More concerning still, a reading of the virology literature confirms that today's science does not have the power to deliver accurate models. Science lacks the most basic understanding about viral transmission, a core input to any epidemiological model of viral spread. A summary of the current state of knowledge is provided in a 2008 paper by Cannell et al.[89] Human studies attempting sick-to-well viral transmission have failed over the past century or more to accurately model influenza transmission "in spite of having numerous acutely ill influenza patients, in various stages of their illness, carefully cough, spit, and breathe on a combined total of >150 well patients." The confidence with which today's epidemiological models assume the trajectory of a respiratory virus is not grounded in scientific reality. Epidemiological models are more accurately seen as a form of speculation, on which it is perilous to build public policy.

---

[87] Levitt, Michael et al (2020). "Predicting the Trajectory of Any COVID19 Epidemic From the Best Straight Line," in *medRxiv* 2020.06.26.20140814; https://archive.ph/vp7Gw.
[88] Michael Levitt explains the difference in structure and behaviour of these functions at http://youtu.be/Uw2ZTaiN97k. Also see Sayers, Freddie (2020), "Nobel prize-winning scientist: the Covid-19 epidemic was never exponential," in *Unherd*, 2 May 2020, https://bit.ly/3ahiJoH.
[89] Cannell, J.J., Zasloff, M., Garland, C.F. et al (2008). "On the epidemiology of influenza," in *Virol J* 5, 29. https://doi.org/10.1186/1743-422X-5-29.

3.3 Twelve principles of public health: Martin Kulldorff

Due to the society-wide impacts of public health interventions, a public health policy-making process that considers multiple dimensions and perspectives is essential.

Epidemiologist and biostatistician Martin Kulldorff has written that good public health policy must satisfy 12 principles:[90]

> 1. Public health is about all health outcomes, not just a single disease like COVID19. It is important to also consider harms from public health measures.
>
> 2. Public health is about the long term rather than the short term. Spring COVID19 lockdowns simply delayed and postponed the pandemic to the fall.
>
> 3. Public health is about everyone. It should not be used to shift the burden of disease from the affluent to the less affluent, as the COVID19 lockdowns have done.
>
> 4. Public health is global. Public health scientists need to consider the global impact of their recommendations.
>
> 5. Risks and harms cannot be completely eliminated, but they can be reduced. Elimination and zero-COVID strategies backfire, making things worse.
>
> 6. Public health should focus on high-risk populations. For COVID19, many standard public health measures were never used to protect high-risk older people, leading to unnecessary deaths.
>
> 7. While contact tracing and isolation is critically important for some infectious diseases, it is futile and counterproductive for common infections such as influenza and COVID19.
>
> 8. A case is only a case if a person is sick. Mass testing asymptomatic individuals is harmful to public health.
>
> 9. Public health is about trust. To gain the trust of the public, public health officials and the media must be honest and trust the public. Shaming and fear should never be used in a pandemic.

---

[90] Tweets dated 19 December 2020 by Martin Kulldorff, https://bit.ly/3wyIQzY.

10. Public health scientists and officials must be honest with what is not known. For example, epidemic models should be run with the whole range of plausible input parameters.

11. In public health, open civilized debate is profoundly critical. Censoring, silencing and smearing leads to fear of speaking, herd thinking and distrust.

12. It is important for public health scientists and officials to listen to the public, who are living the public health consequences. This pandemic has proved that many non-epidemiologists understand public health better than some epidemiologists.

4. Extreme interventions were ruled out by pre-2020 science

In this chapter I review the scientific literature to identify options that were considered suitable pre-2020 for dealing with a COVID-like respiratory pandemic. I proceed from a review of accepted medical principles and laws, through to how these were reflected in the pre-COVID consensus that would merit the appellation of "The Science" before 2020 on managing a respiratory pandemic.

The pre-2020 consensus codified decades of virological and public health science, implying that a huge amount of evidence would be required in order to overturn it. The proof provided of the wisdom of COVID policies in 2020 therefore needed to have been so groundbreaking that it was capable of overturning all prior knowledge in this area. Failure to provide such proof and proceeding regardless to impose a harmful policy shown previously to have failed would constitute a betrayal of good public health and policymaking practice.

4.1 A spectrum of options

Responsible policy analysis considers a range of feasible options. Reflecting this principle, the *User Guide to the Australian Government Guide to Regulatory Impact Analysis* stipulates that "[a] RIS [regulatory impact statement] needs to include at least three options."[91]

A full suite of options to deal with a pandemic like COVID would range across the spectrum from "doing very little, and voluntarily, with a low-cost burden on society" to "doing quite a lot, with some mandatory requirements that impose a high-cost burden." In between would be some mix of voluntary and mandatory requirements.

If this were a prospective CBA, I would consider such a repre-

---

[91] The Office of Best Practice Regulation, Department of Premier and Cabinet, Australian Government (2021). *User Guide to the Australian Government Guide to Regulatory Impact Analysis*, https://archive.ph/I2HUX.

sentative suite of options before selecting one (such as whole-of-population lockdowns and border closures), and I would retain for further consideration only options that pass the basic tests outlined in previous sections. Given the limited scope and retrospective nature of this CBA, however, I do not review the less burdensome options here. The goal of this report is instead to estimate the effects of the high-intervention policy that was actually implemented.

As a precursor to this analysis, I consider in this chapter what lessons can be drawn from pre-COVID government documents and scientific literature in regard to the wisdom of opting for highly burdensome options such as border closures, quarantines, and lockdowns. If such policies had been a good idea, then hundreds of pre-2020 scientific contributions should have recommended them after evaluating their costs and benefits. Instead, according to pre-2020 scientific consensus, such options were considered unreasonable.

4.2 Pre-2020 policy documents ruled out quarantines and lockdowns

4.2.1 *Australia's pandemic plans rule out highly burdensome options*

Workplace closures are only supposed to be a last-resort option and only for "extraordinarily severe pandemics"[92] according to the WHO's 2019 guidelines, which also cautioned that the quality of evidence for such action was "very low." In Australia, highly burdensome policy options of this sort would not have been considered reasonable prior to 2020 for a threat like COVID.

Australia's pandemic plans outline a range of interventions for different levels of pandemic severity. Highly burdensome options like whole-of-population lockdowns are not even listed, having presumably been culled at an early stage during the assessment process.

---

[92] See page 19 of the WHO's October 2019 report, *Non-pharmaceutical public health measures for mitigating the risk and impact of epidemic and pandemic influenza*: https://bit.ly/3yO2No9.

These plans universally take a risk-based approach that implicitly weighs costs and benefits. As an example, Victoria's pandemic plan, the *COVID-19 Pandemic plan for the Victorian Health Sector,*[93] published on 10 March 2020, 'focused on protecting vulnerable Victorians.'

In a similar vein, Australia's COVID pandemic plan[94] classifies pandemics into three categories based on severity. Under Scenario One, "the majority of cases are likely to experience mild to moderate clinical features. People in at-risk groups and those with comorbidities may experience more severe illness." Under Scenario Two, "People in at-risk groups may experience severe illness. As the number of cases grows the number of people presenting for medical care is likely to be higher than for severe seasonal influenza and primary care and hospital services will be under severe pressure, particularly in areas associated with respiratory illness and acute care."

With 898 COVID deaths in Australia in 2020, it is impossible to argue that the hospital system was under any "severe pressure" from COVID. 4090 influenza and pneumonia deaths in Australia in 2019, and commensurate non-fatal influenza and pneumonia cases, were handled without panic or extreme measures. The few tens of thousands of COVID cases that arose in 2020, with only a small proportion of these being treated at hospital, were well within the capacity of Australia's health system to handle. Even if we take a generous approach to the classification of the pandemic – a bias that I conservatively take in this paper, in order to construct the strongest case in favour of the government's narrative and policies – COVID has at most imposed "Scenario Two"-level pressure upon our health system.

4.2.2 *Social distancing measures have limited use*

Prior to 2020, it was widely understood that social distancing measures have only a temporary, modest effect on the spread of patho-

---

[93] Department of Health, Victoria (2020). Website for COVID-19 Pandemic Plan for the Victorian Health Sector. https://bit.ly/3G61X7C.

[94] Department of Health, Australian Government (2020). *Australian Health Sector Emergency Response Plan for Novel Coronavirus (COVID-19)*, https://bit.ly/3wKgOk1.

gens, while causing enormous social, health and economic harm. In 2015, a study reviewed such measures based on actions taken during the 2009 swine flu pandemic.[95] In 2019, an Australian government report summarised this paper's findings.[96] It was thus known within the Australian government that non-pharmaceutical measures like social distancing have limited validity and carry large costs.

4.2.3 *The WHO's pre-2020 position ruled out highly burdensome options*

On 24 January 2020 at the commencement of the Wuhan lockdowns, Gauden Galea, the World Health Organization's representative in China, made it clear that "trying to contain a city of 11 million people is new to science. The lockdown of 11 million people is unprecedented in public health history, so it is certainly not a recommendation the WHO has made."[97]

The October 2019 WHO pandemic guidelines[98] require an assessment of the "balance of benefits and harms" for each intervention, along with other considerations including ethical issues. In addition to workplace closure being "a [possible] last step that is only considered in extraordinarily severe epidemics and pandemics," the guidelines note that contact tracing, quarantine of exposed individuals, border closure and entry and exit screening are "[n]ot recommended under any circumstances."

Thus, the WHO did not recommend lockdowns or other harsh measures as pandemic management policies pre-2020.

[95] Harunor, Rashid et al (2015). "Evidence compendium and advice on social distancing and other related measures for response to an influenza pandemic," in *Paediatric Respiratory Reviews*, Volume 16, Issue 2, March 2015, pp. 119-126, https://pubmed.ncbi.nlm.nih.gov/24630149/.

[96] Department of Health, Australian Government, https://bit.ly/3PFxf9X. This document summarises the evidence presented in Rashid, H. et al (2014), "Evidence compendium and advice on social distancing and other related measures for response to an influenza pandemic," https://pubmed.ncbi.nlm.nih.gov/24630149/.

[97] Senger, Michael P. (2020). "China's Global Lockdown Propaganda Campaign," in *Tablet*, 16 September 2020, https://bit.ly/3yS93eD.

[98] World Health Organisation (2019). *Non-pharmaceutical public health measures for mitigating the risk and impact of epidemic and pandemic influenza*, https://bit.ly/3yO2No9.

4.3 Border closures, lockdowns and quarantines were known not to work

On 24 June 2020, Sweden's State Epidemiologist Anders Tegnell exclaimed at the policies being implemented worldwide: "It was as if the world had gone mad, and everything we had discussed was forgotten."[99] On 29 August 2020, Harvard Medical School Professor Martin Kulldorff summarised why lockdowns do not work: "By increasing other types of morbidity during lockdowns, we end up with much higher mortality in the long-term with lockdowns."[100] This was not news: it was widely understood prior to 2020 in the field of epidemiology.

4.3.1 *Anthony Fauci opposed quarantines and lockdowns prior to 2020*

Anthony Fauci has played a prominent role in designing the 2020 pandemic policies of the USA. The policies he recommended during the COVID pandemic entirely contradict what he previously advocated. For example:

- Quarantines: In 2014, Fauci did not advocate quarantines even for Ebola health workers.[101]

- Shutdowns: As late as 24 January 2020, Fauci expressed opposition to lockdowns, saying "historically when you shut things down it doesn't have a major effect."[102]

4.3.2 *'Disease Mitigation Measures in the Control of Pandemic Influenza'*

A 2006 paper by Thomas V. Inglesby et al (with epidemiologist Donald Henderson as a co-author) rejected "large-scale quarantine"

---

[99] Rolander, Niclas (2020). "Sweden's Covid Expert Says 'World Went Mad' With Lockdowns," in *Bloomberg Quint*, 24 June 2020, https://bit.ly/3PExylo.

[100] Tweet dated 29 August 2020 by Martin Kulldorff, https://archive.ph/PUdp2.

[101] NBC News (2014). "Fauci: Returning Ebola Health Workers Shouldn't Face 'Draconian' Rules," 26 October 2014, https://archive.ph/Sckzc.

[102] CNN (2020). "China is being 'quite transparent', says NIH head," 24 January 2020, https://bit.ly/3PEZDJs.

(lockdowns) to fight influenza on the basis of its extraordinary social costs:

> There are no historical observations or scientific studies that support the confinement by quarantine of groups of possibly infected people for extended periods to slow the spread of influenza. A World Health Organization Writing Group, after reviewing the literature and considering contemporary international experience, concluded that "forced isolation and quarantine are ineffective and impractical." Despite this recommendation by experts, mandatory large-scale quarantine continues to be considered as an option by some authorities and government officials.
>
> The interest in quarantine reflects the views and conditions prevalent more than 50 years ago, when much less was known about the epidemiology of infectious diseases and when there was far less international and domestic travel in a less densely populated world. It is difficult to identify circumstances in the past half-century when large-scale quarantine has been effectively used in the control of any disease. The negative consequences of large-scale quarantine are so extreme (forced confinement of sick people with the well; complete restriction of movement of large populations; difficulty in getting critical supplies, medicines, and food to people inside the quarantine zone) that this mitigation measure should be eliminated from serious consideration.[103]

Implicit in this assessment is a cost-benefit analysis concluding that the negative consequences of large-scale quarantine implemented supposedly to fight infectious disease are not only "extreme," but higher than their limited benefits, and that therefore that a policy of lockdowns is unwise.

In 2007, epidemiologist Donald Henderson made the need for a cost-benefit test even more explicit. In relation to social distancing interventions, in 2007, he 'cautioned against relying on models that

---

[103] Inglesby, Thomas V., et al (2006). "Disease Mitigation Measures in the Control of Pandemic Influenza," in *Biosecurity and Bioterrorism*. Volume 4, Number 4, 2006, https://pubmed.ncbi.nlm.nih.gov/17238820/.

do not take into consideration the adverse effects or practical constraints that such public health interventions would entail. Accepting such models uncritically, he warned, could result in policies that "take a perfectly manageable epidemic and turn it into a national disaster".[104]

4.3.3 The index case problem

Donald Henderson was a major figure in epidemiology and public health who was instrumental in eradicating smallpox from the planet. Henderson's work shows that the spread of most viruses cannot be stopped unless the first case (the "index case") in a country is stopped, and the next such index case is stopped, and so on for every subsequent index case.[105] He notes that some viruses can indeed be controlled through quarantines of the sick, and successful attempts have been made to do so (e.g., for Ebola). By contrast, for most viruses, including the flu, if even a single person who may not have obvious symptoms slips through the net of control, the battle is lost. It is far more sensible in such cases, Henderson observed, not to implement hard controls on human movement but rather to manage the disease in order to minimise harm. In his words, expressed during a panel discussion on March 5, 2010 at a conference entitled "The 2009 H1N1 Experience: Policy Implications for Future Infectious Disease Emergencies:"[106]

> In the smallpox program there were the questions: What do we do about screening people?
>
> And this was something we were really deeply concerned about with smallpox.

---

[104] Institute of Medicine (US) Forum on Microbial Threats. Ethical and Legal Considerations in Mitigating Pandemic Disease: Workshop Summary (2007). Washington (DC): National Academies Press (US); Summary and Assessment, https://www.ncbi.nlm.nih.gov/books/NBK54157/.

[105] See Henderson's comments on this topic from timestamp 32:35 on a panel at the 5 March 2010 conference on "The 2009 H1N1 experience: policy implications for future infectious disease emergencies," at http://youtu.be/8rEV857R0LE ("Role of Disease Containment in Control of Epidemics (Panel)").

[106] See from timestamp 33:55 at http://youtu.be/8rEV857R0LE.

And so, we went into the records rather thoroughly since about 1945. And there are about just under 50 importations of smallpox that could be well-documented.

And the question is: How many might we have intercepted who might have had just fever or rash?

And the fact was none.

So, anything we were doing at a border crossing to try to interrupt smallpox coming across the border would have been quite futile.

I then had some discussions with our CDC colleagues and the quarantine group down there and thought about this. I thought, you know, as I said to them, CDC investigates a lot of different outbreaks, and many of these you can tell which are the first case [the index case], and so forth. It'd be interesting to see how many instances we could identify in which that first individual might have been intercepted coming into the country.

And I'm still waiting for one example so far.

I think the point is that this idea that in this day and age one is going to intercept people coming across the border and you're going to stop the spread of the disease is a concept that was antiquated a very long time ago.

4.3.4 *International travel may reduce the chance of lethal pandemics*

Since at least since her "Princeton in Europe" lecture in 2013, Dr Sunetra Gupta of Oxford University has been expounding a revolutionary theory about pathogenic spread:

Virulent pathogens cannot be the only things we bring back from the countries where they've originated. It is more likely that we're constantly importing less virulent forms which go undetected because they're asymptomatic and these may well have the effect of attenuating the severity of infection with their more virulent cousins.

After all the oldest trick up our sleeves is, as vaccination goes, is to use a milder species to protect against a more virulent species. Perhaps this is something we're inadvertently achieving by mixing more widely with a variety of international pathogens.[107]

This theory is based on the same principle that applies to children, who "benefit from being exposed to this (covid) and other seasonal coronaviruses."[108] Getting a less harmful infection protects children against more serious infections in the future. The T cells in our immune system are stimulated and activated by weaker viruses. Dr Gupta believes on this basis that "the best way to [safeguard against pandemics] is to build up a global wall of immunity. And it may be that we're unwittingly achieving this through our current patterns of international travel."

As Sunetra Gupta wrote along with Thompson et al in 2018, "Not only does cross-immunity protect individuals from infection, but our results also suggest that cross-immunity might be a potential explanatory factor as to why there has not been a pandemic as devastating as the 1918 influenza epidemic in the century since, despite the emergence of a strain antigenically similar to the 1918 pandemic strain in 2009."[109]

On this basis one might hypothesise that it is unlikely, given the mass-scale international travel that has become the norm over the past few decades, that humanity would experience a very significant respiratory pandemic again. Consistent with this hypothesis, COVID has turned out to be a modest pandemic by historical and pathogenic comparison.

The logic above implies that the steep and prolonged decline in international travel after the emergence of COVID may have in-

---

[107] http://youtu.be/kclL0F985DYh ("Sunetra Gupta showed in 2013 how international travel eliminates the prospect of a major pandemic").

[108] *Evening Standard* (2020). "The Londoner: Let children be exposed to viruses, says Professor Gupta," 2 September 2020. https://bit.ly/3yR4MYJ.

[109] Thompson et al (2019). "Increased frequency of travel in the presence of cross-immunity may act to decrease the chance of a global pandemic," in *Philosophical Transactions of Royal Society B* (Biological Sciences), 6 May 2019. https://doi.org/10.1098/rstb.2018.0274

creased the risk posed by future infectious pathogens to the Australian population, and particularly to those most vulnerable, such as our elderly.[110]

4.3.5 Why do lockdowns cause harm?

Locked-down nations focus their energy on trying to prevent people at low risk (such as the young) from contracting the virus. This focus has many harmful effects. Most obviously, it leaves fewer resources for the government to deploy to cocoon and care for the old and sick who are most at risk. As a result, more of the truly vulnerable may die in locked-down nations.[111] Imposing crippling restrictions on a large fraction of the population ostensibly to reduce harms which might be experienced by a very small fraction of the population – even if those restrictions were successful in achieving the proposed ends – may logically cause significant net harm. Through what sorts of mechanisms is this harm caused?

First, lockdowns slow the development of immunity among the healthy who therefore cannot act as barriers to the further spread of disease. In the typical trajectory leading to high levels of immunity to a respiratory virus, as the popular "Susceptible, Infected, Recovered" models aim to reflect,[112] population infection levels peak fairly quickly and those who have recovered become immune, which then makes it harder for the virus to continue to spread to others.

---

[110] To be conservative, I omit this possible dimension of damage from the costs caused by lockdowns estimated in the present report.

[111] In Victoria, for example, the government was doing so many disparate things that affected everyone, instead of focusing on protecting the vulnerable, that insufficient numbers of high-quality masks were provided to healthcare and aged care workers, who promptly caught COVID and passed it on to the vulnerable (see https://archive.ph/HAHMG – ABC news 10 July 2020: "Victorian healthcare workers continue to face shortages of PPE as coronavirus cases ramp up"). This partly explains why so many elderly Victorians residing in aged care homes succumbed in the first wave in 2020. Aged care director and union leader Carolyn Smith describes the inadequate resources devoted towards the protection and treatment of our high-risk people in a video in August 2020: https://archive.ph/8cIrn.

[112] For a short introduction to such models, see Okabe, Yutaka et al (2020), "A Mathematical Model of Epidemics – A Tutorial for Students," in *Mathematics* 2020, 8(7), 1174, https://doi.org/10.3390/math8071174.

Second, lockdowns force people indoors and away from broader society, resulting in a higher chance of a poorer immune response if infection occurs, for example via vitamin D insufficiency and stress, and a higher chance of viral transmission within the home. Third, lockdowns have been found to increase unhealthy habits like poor exercise and dietary choices, which may further depress the immune response. Obesity, for example, increases the risk of being hospitalised with COVID.[113] CSIRO survey-based research[114] has shown that 2 in 5 respondents gained weight during lockdowns, while over 66% of respondents reported that lockdowns negatively affected exercise. In many ways, lockdowns also make it more difficult for ill or injured people to receive care for problems other than COVID (such as diabetes), thus exacerbating their COVID risk through increased co-morbidity.

Through such mechanisms, lockdowns can raise the risk not only of additional COVID deaths and suffering but of death and suffering from a wide range of other causes.

4.4 Actual policy choices

What did governments in Australia and the world actually do, against the backdrop of scientific knowledge sketched above? Many, including Australia, chose lockdowns.

Around the world, countries that seemed to avoid a first wave of COVID initially simply had one later on. Australia's case is reasonably consistent with this overall pattern, although being an island nation has affected our experience. Australia's governments were unable to create a perfect shield, and the pattern of COVID deaths in the country shows some similarity to other nations (Figure 4.1), except that the aggressive attempts at suppression via international border closures probably postponed some COVID deaths.

---

[113] https://www.thelancet.com/journals/landia/article/PIIS2213-8587(20)30274-6/fulltext, "Obesity and COVID-19: Blame isn't a strategy," in *The Lancet Diabetes & Endocrinology*, 7 August 2020 editorial.
[114] CSIRO (2020). "CSIRO study reveals COVID-19's impact on weight and emotional wellbeing," 16 June 2020, https://bit.ly/3MwFjYB.

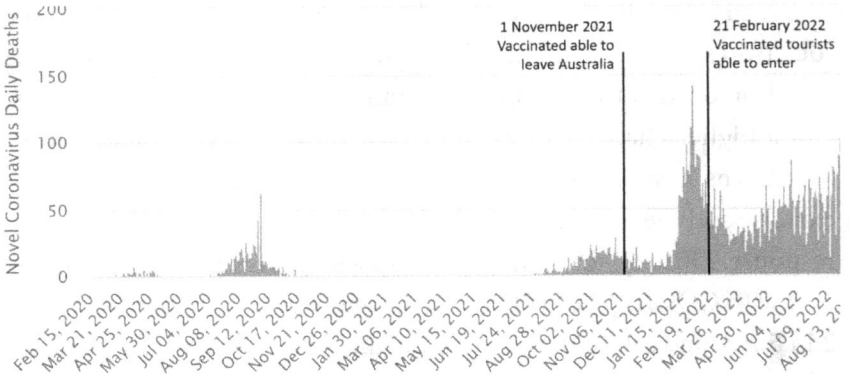

Figure 4.1: Daily number of reported COVID deaths in Australia[115]

In my book *The Great Covid Panic* (2021) with Paul Frijters and Michael Baker, I categorise countries and regions of the world based on the policy options with which they responded to the COVID pandemic. We used the Oxford Covid-19 Government Response Tracker to estimate stringency.

- The first were the **Minimalists,** like South Dakota in the USA, that followed standard pandemic plans. Such places saw similar numbers of COVID cases to their neighbours, while life went on almost as normally as is possible in a major recession.

- The second were the **Pragmatists** which include countries like Sweden, Korea, Japan, Taiwan, Iceland and Estonia (although some would argue that Sweden falls under the Minimalist category). These countries implemented different policies than would be taken in normal times to address a respiratory virus like COVID, including in some cases widespread testing and targeted restrictions and masks, but stopped short of extended wholesale lockdowns.

- The final group, comprising around 90% of the world's population, were the **Covid Cults**. The Covid Cult group comprised most of Europe and the Americas, Southeast Asia, India, China,

---

[115] *Source*: Worldometer, https://www.worldometers.info/coronavirus/country/australia/, extracted on 8 April 2022.

Australia, New Zealand and much of Africa. Covid Cult governments were usually quick to implement lockdowns, with little to no input from experts offering alternative data or holding alternative views. The public discourse that typically precedes major policy decisions in democracies was cast aside in Covid Cult regions, under the pretext that leaders needed to act quickly and decisively.

Over time, Covid Cult governments changed their objective from 'flattening the curve' to eliminating the virus, a transformation that necessitated stronger suppression of dissent and the tightening or extending of restrictions. These countries suffered enormous collateral damage, widespread abuse of power, and mass invasion of privacy. Their governments periodically acknowledged the existence of the damage being done to their own countries, but still initiated a fresh cycle of draconian measures when new waves of COVID arrived. They adhered to the narrative that the future depended on sacrificing the present.

In the book we plot the COVID fatality data for these three groups of countries from 1 January 2020 to 25 July 2021 and find that (globally) the Covid Cult nations had consistently higher reported COVID deaths than the Pragmatists. There was no extraordinary wave of deaths among countries that did not lock down for long periods of time. Politicians' claims notwithstanding, it was evidently possible to have minimal restrictions and also minimal numbers of COVID deaths, and the reasons for those low death numbers might well have been entirely unrelated to policy choices, such as having a population with high prior immunity or relatively few vulnerable old people.

The vast bulk of COVID deaths in all three groups of countries occurred between late 2020 and mid-2021, so fully 9 months after most of the lockdowns began, in March-April 2020. This immediately makes a mockery of the idea that lockdowns were preventing bad outcomes, and instead raises the question of how they may have in fact increased the number of COVID deaths.

Australia's cult-like obsession with COVID is best illustrated in the experience of Melbourne. This city experienced the longest and some of the most restrictive lockdowns seen in the world. Reuters reported that by 21 October 2021, Melbourne had "spent a cumulative 262 days, or nearly nine months, under stay-home orders since March 2020 - the world's longest, exceeding a 234-day lockdown in Buenos Aires."[116] Even when the lockdowns were declared to have ended in Melbourne, there was no quick return to normalcy. The obsession with COVID continued still across Australia even into 2022. For example, on 29 October 2021, Queensland confirmed that it would not open its domestic borders with the rest of Australia until at least January 2022, and indeed that promise was fulfilled.[117]

One could be forgiven for thinking that Australia's governments remained, even in late 2021, at least mentally committed to "zero COVID" despite this being explicitly contraindicated by law. As Section 5 of Part 1 of Chapter 1 of the *Biosecurity Act 2015* specifies:[118]

[The] Appropriate Level of Protection (ALOP) for Australia against biosecurity risks is a high level of sanitary and phytosanitary protection aimed at reducing biosecurity risks to a very low level, but not to zero.

[116] Reuters (2021). "Melbourne readies to exit world's longest COVID-19 lockdown," 21 October 2021, https://bit.ly/3wBboJe.
[117] "Deputy Premier Steven Miles has revealed the hard state border will not ease until January at the earliest," https://bit.ly/3MFlNsV.
[118] https://www.legislation.gov.au/Details/C2020C00127.

5. Brief review of the COVID-era cost-benefit literature on lockdowns

In this chapter I outline the literature and opinions aired since the emergence of COVID by epidemiologists, scientists and economists about the costs and benefits of lockdowns. Despite a vast amount of pro-lockdown contributions, including by a large number of scientists and economists, the views expressed by many independent scientists since the emergence of COVID have aligned with the consensus of pre-2020 science.

To motivate this review, a selection of the many pro-lockdown contributions in Australia is listed below in chronological order.

- **17 March 2020:** Almost 2,500 doctors led by Dr Hemant Garg send a letter to Minister Greg Hunt, demanding lockdown.[119]

- **22 March 2020:** Roger Bradbury, Emeritus Professor at the Australian National University's Crawford School of Public Policy, demands total lockdown.[120]

- **24 March 2020:** Over 5000 doctors led by Dr Greg Kelly sign an open letter to the Prime Minister about tougher lockdown measures.[121]

- **30 March 2020**: A paper by C. Raina MacIntyre (UNSW), Louisa Jorm (UNSW), Richard Nunes-Vaz (Flinders University), and Timothy Churches (UNSW) demands a short, sharp lockdown.[122]

---

[119] Nelson, Felicity (2020), "Doctors urge government to shut everything down," in *Medical Republic*, 17 March 2020, https://bit.ly/3lEwkIQ.

[120] Bradbury, Roger (2020). "Why we need to lock everything down," in *Financial Review*, 22 March 2020, https://bit.ly/3Pz6Dr9.

[121] *Sydney Morning Herald* (2020). "Thousands of doctors sign petition calling for national lockdown now," 24 March 2020, https://bit.ly/3MGDRmD; also discussed here: *Women's Agenda* (2020), "An open letter to the PM from Australian doctors is circulating," 16 March 2020, https://bit.ly/38ckK4Q.

[122] University of New South Wales, Centre for Research Excellence Integrated Systems for Epidemic Response (2020). "Regaining Control: The Case For A Short, Sharp Lockdown (Rather Than The Slow Trickle We've Had So Far)," https://bit.ly/3Gd2k0w.

- **19 April 2020**: An open letter is released, signed by 256 economists, in support of lockdowns.[123]

- **13 October 2020**: It is reported that "top Australian epidemiologists Professor James McCaw and Professor Catherine Bennett have cautioned that key measures must be in place before lockdowns can be eased."[124]

- **27 July 2021**: A UNSW BusinessThink blog featuring Richard Holden and John Quiggin is published noting that "A clear majority of economists surveyed by The Conversation in May 2020 (after the end of the national lockdown) supported strong social distancing measures to keep R below 1."[125]

- **13 September 2021**: OzSAGE advocates for the re-imposition of restrictions, allegedly because NSW's ICU beds would be full over Christmas: "reopening the state once 70 per cent of people aged 16 and over are fully vaccinated may lead to all the state's intensive care unit beds being full for five weeks over Christmas and almost 1000 people dying from COVID-19."[126]

- **21 September 2021**: University of Melbourne researchers release a report entitled "2022 will be better: COVID-19 Pandemic Tradeoffs modelling." Newspaper coverage of the report notes that "Australians will still need to endure lockdowns for at least half the year even once 80 per cent of adults are fully vaccinated against Covid-19."[127]

None of these contributions incorporated a robust cost-benefit

---

[123] An Open Letter by Australian Economists on Tradeoffs During the COVID-19 Crisis, http://covid19openletter.net/.

[124] Hendrie, Doug (2020). "Renewed calls to end lockdown rejected by RACGP and other experts," in *NewsGP*, The Royal Australian College of General Practitioners (RACGP), 13 October 2020, https://bit.ly/3sMoh0I.

[125] Holden, Richard (2021). "Why most economists continue to back lockdowns," in *Business Think*, University of New South Wales, 27 July 2021, https://bit.ly/3sRQAL8.

[126] *WA Today* (2021). "As it happened: Digital pass to allow vaccinated Australians to travel; hospitals under pressure as NSW, Victorian COVID-19 cases rise," 14 September 2021, https://bit.ly/3Ntxz9Y.

[127] Chang, Charis (2021). "Long lockdowns still needed to keep Covid-19 cases down despite vaccinations, new modelling suggests," in News.com.au, 21 September 2021, https://bit.ly/3MGEsVp.

analysis recognising the many types of human costs directly caused by lockdowns.

The chapters about crowds and brainwashing, the dynamics of power, and the corruption of science in my co-authored book, *The Great Covid Panic*, provide a fuller explanation as to why so many scientists and journalists supported lockdowns in response to COVID.

5.1 Expert opinions on the net costs of lockdowns

On 20 May 2020, Michael Levitt, a Nobel Prize winner in chemistry who has spent considerable time looking at COVID pandemic data, stated:

> There is no doubt in my mind, that when we come to look back on this, the damage done by lockdown will exceed any saving of lives by a huge factor.[128]

Professor John Ioannidis wrote on 3 June 2020 that "[m]assacres in overwhelmed hospitals with contaminated personnel and in nursing homes represent the lion's share of deaths. Hospital preparedness, universal personnel screening, draconian infection control, and social distancing in these locations are indispensable. However, blind lockdown of entire populations has questionable added benefits."[129] Core to his argument were the facts that the infection fatality rate of COVID was far lower than initially estimated, and that risk varied substantially across individuals.

Dr David Nabarro, Britain's envoy to the World Health Organisation, said on 10 October 2020 that lockdowns were causing a 'ghastly global catastrophe:'[130]

---

[128] Stringham, E.P. (2020). "Nobel Laureate Michael Levitt on the Lockdowns: 'I think it is a huge mistake,'" in American Institute for Economic Research, 31 May 2020, https://bit.ly/3Ns9YGz.

[129] Melnick, E.R. and Ioannidis, J.P.A. (2020). "Should governments continue lockdown to slow the spread of covid-19?" in *BMJ*; 369:m1924 doi:10.1136/bmj.m1924, 3 June 2020, https://www.bmj.com/content/369/bmj.m1924.

[130] *Daily Mail* (2020). "'STOP locking-down to control Covid': Britain's WHO envoy pleads with world leaders to stop using lockdowns as their 'primary' means of tackling virus because it is 'doubling' global poverty," 10 October 2020, https://bit.ly/3MFFD7u.

'We in the World Health Organisation do not advocate lockdowns as a primary means of controlling this virus,' Dr Nabarro said. 'The only time we believe a lockdown is justified is to buy you time to reorganise, regroup, rebalance your resources, protect your health workers who are exhausted. But by and large, we'd rather not do it.'

Pointing to lockdown impacts he noted, 'it seems we may well have a doubling of world poverty by next year. We may well have at least a doubling of child malnutrition because children are not getting meals at school and their parents, in poor families, are not able to afford it.'

'This is a terrible, ghastly global catastrophe, actually. And so, we really do appeal to all world leaders: stop using lockdown as your primary control method.'

In *Newsweek* on 30 October 2020, Professors Martin Kulldorff, Sunetra Gupta and Jay Bhattacharya summarised the effect of lockdowns across the world:

> Lockdown strategies have led to many avoidable deaths among those at high risk from COVID-19 infections, while creating enormous collateral non-COVID health damage on everyone else.[131]

5.2 Comparing locked down and non-locked down regions

Some scientists and economists have conducted comparisons of similarly placed regions to gauge the impact of lockdowns.

5.2.1 Comparison of "early lockdown" and "late lockdown" European nations

In March 2021, epidemiologist Dr Raghib Ali compared countries with early lockdowns to those with late lockdowns. He found either no difference between them in endpoint COVID outcomes, or that nations that locked down earlier ended up with more deaths:

> Based on current trends, it seems likely that many of these

---

[131] Martin Kulldorff, Sunetra Gupta and Jay Bhattacharya (2020). "We Should Focus on Protecting the Vulnerable from COVID Infection," in *NewsWeek,* 30 October 2020, https://bit.ly/38BLaNL.

countries that we thought were doing well due to their early lockdowns and small first waves will end up having higher excess mortality than the UK, including Czechia, Poland, Portugal, and many others ... On the so called two-week 'circuit breaker lockdowns,' it should also be remembered that Wales did follow SAGE's advice – but ended up with the same level of infections and deaths as England as it just postponed more infections to the winter months.[132]

In his words, one reason why many nations that implemented early lockdowns ended up with even more total COVID deaths is that "by effectively delaying part of the first wave from the spring until the second wave in the winter, this meant that many countries had a higher proportion of the population still susceptible to infection, and so led to even higher death tolls as health systems struggled to cope."

A July 2021 analysis by Martin Lally of 33 European countries[133] found that more stringent policies in terms of lockdowns and border restrictions did not lead to fewer deaths:

Regressing the death rate per 1m (D) up to 31 December [2020] on the maximum Stringency Index value (S), the population density (PD, in millions per 1,000 square miles), and date of first death (FD, in days from 15 February) yields the following result:

$D = 273.9 + 7.34S + 473.1PD - 12.3FD$

The R^2 is 0.29, and the p values are 0.66, 0.27, 0.10 and 0.10 respectively. The coefficient on S is statistically insignificant and the sign on it is 'wrong' (positive rather than negative).

Lally opines that "lockdowns induce some behaviours that increase the death rate, such as young people returning to live with their older parents, due to loss of their job or closure of the university

[132] Ali, Raghib (2021). "Would an earlier lockdown really have saved tens of thousands of lives?" in *The Telegraph*, 21 March 2021, https://bit.ly/39HxoJq.
[133] Lally, Martin (2021). "The Costs and Benefits of Covid-19 Lockdowns in New Zealand," in *medRxiv* 21 July 2021, 2021.07.15.21260606; doi: 27 July 2021. https://doi.org/10.1101/2021.07.15.21260606.

they were attending, and if already infected to thereby infect their parents, who are at much greater risk of death."

5.2.2 *Worldometer: Tracking results across countries and over time*

A comparative analysis of COVID deaths per million on Worldometer shows that 55 countries including the UK, Italy, France, and the US have experienced a higher death rate with COVID than Sweden, which largely followed risk-based, voluntary policies.[134] This is despite many factors that would make one predict higher COVID deaths in Sweden than in other countries. The dry tinder effect – i.e., lower than normal flu deaths in 2019 – was in effect in 2020, but also, in comparison with the rest of the world's averages, Sweden has an unusually large elderly population: over 5% of its population is over 80, compared with less than 2% globally. Further, at its latitude vitamin D deficiency is prevalent, particularly among dark-skinned residents.[135] Also, many of its aged care centres and nursing homes are high-density establishments,[136] making them particularly vulnerable to the spread of infectious disease.

If lockdowns worked, then this comparatively good performance of Sweden would be highly unlikely. Instead, with its policies, Sweden should have had one of the highest COVID death rates in the world.

5.2.3 *Comparison of Sweden with the UK*

Figure 5.1 compares COVID deaths in the UK and Sweden. These data are consistent with the estimate of Lally,[137] namely that countries with more stringent restrictions ended up with more COVID

---

[134] https://www.worldometers.info/coronavirus/#countries, as at 3 July 2022.

[135] Wandell, Per et al (2018). "Vitamin D deficiency was common in all patients at a Swedish primary care centre, but more so in patients born outside of Europe," in *Z Gesundh Wiss*. 2018; 26(6): 649–652, 27 March 2018, https://www.ncbi.nlm.nih.gov/pmc/articles/PMC6245030/.

[136] E.g., the Berga Vård & Omsorgsboende retirement home in Stockholm, https://reut.rs/36CAOvM.

[137] Lally, Martin (2021). "The Costs and Benefits of Covid-19 Lockdowns in New Zealand," in *medRxiv* 21 July 2021, 2021.07.15.21260606; doi: 27 July 2021. https://doi.org/10.1101/2021.07.15.21260606.

deaths than those with less stringent restrictions, or at best that stringency made no difference. The tally of non-COVID excess deaths also seems to be higher in some nations that imposed stringent lockdowns, although more research is needed to understand the causal factors behind these deaths.[138]

New deaths attributed to Covid-19 in England and Sweden
Seven-day rolling average of new deaths (per 100k)

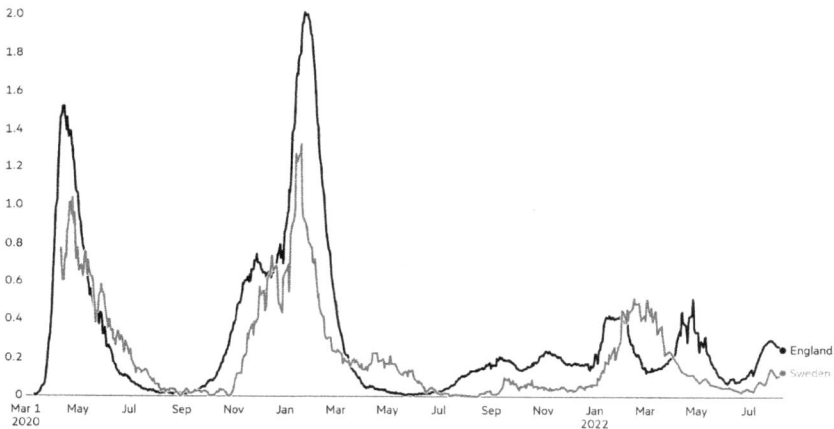

Figure 5.1: Comparison of COVID deaths by 28 June 2022 in the UK and Sweden[139]

5.2.4 *Comparison of states in USA*

South Dakota (population 0.885 million) did not have lockdowns. North Dakota (0.762 million) did. Their COVID death outcomes,

---

[138] It appears from a July 2021 study that while island nations like New Zealand which implemented strong international border controls had lower reported excess deaths during the study period, some large nations which implemented stringent lockdowns had a higher proportion of non-COVID excess deaths than countries with fewer restrictions (e.g., the USA, with 23% extra non-COVID deaths, compares poorly to Sweden, which had no lockdowns and only 4% extra non-COVID deaths, in 2020 (source: https://jamanetwork.com/journals/jamanetworkopen/fullarticle/2781968)). A recent WHO report also documents more excess deaths in the US and in the UK per population than in Sweden in the years 2020 and 2021 (World Health Organization (2022). Global excess deaths associated with COVID-19, January 2020-December 2021, https://bit.ly/3wK0aAR). More research is needed in this area.
[139] Source: https://bit.ly/39NgysM. Updated chart dated 20 May 2022 at: https://bit.ly/3wBtpac.

however, were almost identical: South Dakota's COVID death rate was 2,526 per million, while North Dakota's COVID death rate was 2,312 per million. At a minimum, North Dakota subjected itself to a lot of pain for very little apparent gain.

Many other comparisons have been done, such as between Florida and other states. These studies have found that states with lower restrictions either outperformed more restrictive states, or at least did comparably well, in terms of COVID outcomes.[140]

5.3 Illustrative academic papers examining the impact of the 2020 lockdowns

A vast number of scholars have studied the impacts of the 2020 lockdowns, either in terms of the narrowly stated terms of reference under which they were initially introduced (i.e., to lessen COVID deaths and suffering) or in terms of their broader health outcomes and/or other socioeconomic outcomes.[141] These include:

- In <u>April 2020</u>, T.J. Rogers and colleagues reported the result of a study in which they calculated "a simple one-variable correlation of deaths per million and days to shutdown," where "'days to shutdown' was the time after a state crossed the 1 per million threshold until it ordered businesses shut down." These authors found that "[t]he correlation coefficient was 5.5% [sic: r = -0.055] – so low that the engineers I used to employ would have summarized it as "no correlation" and moved on to find the real cause of the problem. (The trendline sloped downward – states that delayed more tended to have lower death rates – but that's also a meaningless result due to the low correlation coefficient.)."[142] On 20 <u>May 2020</u>, Elaine He at Bloomberg reported "there's little

---

[140] E.g., http://youtu.be/_DOwDAbibQI ("Ivor Cummins: Florida Wins the Science War – Hands Down – no problemo!!!").

[141] A compilation of more than 400 such studies: Alexander, Paul E. (2021). "More Than 400 Studies on the Failure of Compulsory Covid Interventions," Brownstone Institute, 30 November 2021, https://archive.ph/WdAok.

[142] Rodgers, T.J. (2020). "Do Lockdowns Save Many Lives? In Most Places, the Data Say No," in *Wall Street Journal*, 26 April 2020, https://bit.ly/3MG3HXE.

correlation between the severity of a nation's restrictions and whether it managed to curb excess fatalities."[143]

- A <u>June 2020</u> study published in *Advance* by Stefan Homburg and Christof Kuhbandner found that the data "strongly suggests" that "the UK lockdown was both superfluous (it did not prevent an otherwise explosive behavior of the spread of the coronavirus) and ineffective (it did not slow down the death growth rate visibly)."[144]

- In a <u>1 August 2020</u> cross-country study published in *The Lancet*, Rabail Chaudhry et al concluded that "[r]apid border closures, full lockdowns, and wide-spread testing were not associated with COVID-19 mortality per million people."[145]

- In an <u>August 2020</u> National Bureau of Economic Research working paper, authors Andrew Atkeson et al. found that COVID deaths followed a similar pattern "virtually everywhere in the world" and that "[f]ailing to account for this familiar pattern risks overstating the importance of policy mandated NPIs for shaping the progression of this deadly pandemic."[146]

- On <u>29 September 2020</u> *The Australian* reported on a new publication from the Institute of Public Affairs estimating that the "cost of trying to eliminate the coronavirus from Australia is more than annual government spending on defence, education, health and social security combined…From June this year to the middle of 2022, the "elimination strategy" being pursued by state and federal governments will cost $319bn, equivalent to 23 per cent of

[143] He, Elaine (2020). "The Results of Europe's Lockdown Experiment Are In," in Bloomberg, 20 May 2020, https://bit.ly/3MIqP8e.

[144] Homburg, Stefan et al (2020). "Comment on Flaxman et al (2020): The illusory effects of non-pharmaceutical interventions on COVID-19 in Europe," in Advance, 18 June 2020, https://bit.ly/3lxyY39.

[145] https://www.thelancet.com/journals/eclinm/article/PIIS2589-5370(20)30208-X/fulltext, Chaudhry, Rabail et al (2020), "A country level analysis measuring the impact of government actions, country preparedness and socioeconomic factors on COVID-19 mortality and related health outcomes," in eClinicalMedicine, 21 July.

[146] Atkeson, Andrew et al (2020). "Four Stylized Facts about COVID-19," NBER Working Paper 27719, http://www.nber.org/papers/w27719.

GDP, according to the report, *Medical Capacity: An Alternative to Lockdowns.*"[147]

- On 14 October 2020 Jan M. Brauner et al concluded in their preprint study, "The effectiveness of eight nonpharmaceutical interventions against COVID-19 in 41 countries,"[148] that "closing schools and universities was highly effective; that banning gatherings and closing high-risk businesses was effective, but closing most other businesses had limited further benefit; and that many countries may have been able to reduce R below 1 without issuing a stay-at-home order." The paper was later published.

- On 19 November 2020 a paper by De Larochelambert et al[149,149] found that "[s]tringency of the measures settled to fight pandemia, including lockdown, did not appear to be linked with death rate" and that other factors outside governments' short-term control were mainly what drove COVID death rates, such as prevailing life expectancy, co-morbidities, and latitude: "[r]egarding government's actions (i.e., containment and stringency index), no association was found with the outcome, suggesting that the other studied factors were more important in the Covid-19 mortality than political measures implemented to fight the virus, except for the economic support index."

- On 24 December 2020, Eran Bendavid et al noted the following in their study, "Assessing mandatory stay-at-home and business closure effects on the spread of COVID:"

  [W]e fail to find strong evidence supporting a role for more restrictive NPIs in the control of COVID in early 2020. We do not question the role of all public health interventions, or

---

[147] Creighton, Adam (2020). "Coronavirus: Elimination strategy 'will cost us $319bn,'" in *The Australian*, 29 September 2020, https://bit.ly/2ELCrcP. The IPA report itself is available at: https://bit.ly/3ySZVGv.

[148] Brauner, Jan M. et al (2020). "Inferring the effectiveness of government interventions against COVID-19," in *Science*, Vol 371, Issue 6531, 15 December 2020, https://www.science.org/doi/10.1126/science.abd9338.

[149] De Larochelambert, Quentin et al (2020). "Covid-19 Mortality: A Matter of Vulnerability Among Nations Facing Limited Margins of Adaptation," in *Frontiers of Public Health*, 19 November 2020, https://doi.org/10.3389/fpubh.2020.604339.

of coordinated communications about the epidemic, but we fail to find an additional benefit of stay-at-home orders and business closures. The data cannot fully exclude the possibility of some benefits. However, even if they exist, these benefits may not match the numerous harms of these aggressive measures. More targeted public health interventions that more effectively reduce transmissions may be important for future epidemic control without the harms of highly restrictive measures.[150]

- <u>5 February 2021</u>: In their paper, "The impact of non-pharmaceutical interventions on SARS-CoV-2 transmission across 130 countries and territories,"[151] Yang Liu et al concluded that "[e]vidence about the effectiveness of … (stay-at home requirements, public information campaigns, public transport closure, international travel controls, testing, contact tracing) was inconsistent and inconclusive."

- <u>June 2021</u>: Virat Agarwal et al[152] examined 43 countries and all US states, looking for a positive link between shelter-in-place ("SIP") orders and excess deaths. The only countries in which they observed a fall in the trajectory of excess deaths were Australia, New Zealand and Malta. "All three countries are islands," they observed. "In every other country, we observe either no visual change in excess deaths or increases in excess deaths."

Agarwal's June 2021 paper only counts excess deaths in the immediate period around lockdowns. Lockdowns also carry immediate costs of suffering, such as declines in mental health due to loneliness, and long-run costs in many dimensions, which only a complete cost-benefit analysis can reveal.

---

[150] Bendavid, Eran et al (2020). "Assessing mandatory stay-at-home and business closure effects on the spread of COVID-19," in *European Journal of Clinical Investigation*, 24 December 2020, https://onlinelibrary.wiley.com/doi/epdf/10.1111/eci.13484.

[151] Liu, Yang et al (2021). "The impact of non-pharmaceutical interventions on SARS-CoV-2 transmission across 130 countries and territories," in *BMC Medicine*, 5 February 2021, https://archive.ph/vKPMD.

[152] Agrawal, Virat et al (2021). "The impact of the Covid-19 pandemic and policy responses on excess mortality," NBER Working Paper 28930, DOI 10.3386/w28930, http://www.nber.org/papers/w28930.

5.4 Cost-benefit analyses of the 2020 lockdowns

There are a number of ways to undertake a cost-benefit analysis. A useful summary of methods is provided by Paul Frijters in the *Vienna Yearbook of Population Research*.[153] Different authors inevitably use different methods and currencies, and include different factors in their analysis. Data shortcomings, which are inevitable, also add to the lack of direct comparability of the methods or outcomes of most CBAs.

This diversity has a compelling advantage. When different CBAs conducted by independent researchers taking different, yet careful and broadly reasonable, approaches arrive at a similar basic conclusion, then the strength of that conclusion is enhanced. In the case of COVID lockdowns, many scholars have conducted CBAs of lockdown policies, and in the main, these assessments have concluded that lockdowns are harmful on net and therefore not a good policy option. In science, this is what we would term a robust finding.

A few of the many CBAs of lockdown policies that have been undertaken across the world are outlined below.

5.4.1 *Douglas Allen's September 2021 CBA for Canada, and review of over 100 CBAs*

On 29 September 2021, Douglas Allen, Professor of Economics at Simon Fraser University, published a review of 100 cost-benefit analyses of the COVID lockdowns – most of which he found to have significant shortcomings. He then prepared his own analysis of lockdowns in Canada, and found that the costs of lockdowns exceeded their benefits by a factor of 141:

> An examination of over 100 Covid-19 studies reveals that many relied on false assumptions that over-estimated the benefits and under-estimated the costs of lockdown. The most recent research has shown that lockdowns have had, at best, a marginal effect on the number of Covid-19 deaths.

---

[153] Frijters, Paul (2021). "WELLBYs, cost-benefit analyses and the Easterlin Discount," in *Vienna Yearbook of Population Research* (Vol.19), pp. 1-26.

Generally speaking, the ineffectiveness stemmed from individual changes in behavior: either non-compliance or behavior that mimicked lockdowns. The limited effectiveness of lockdowns explains why, after more than one year, the unconditional cumulative Covid-19 deaths per million is not negatively correlated with the stringency of lockdown across countries. Using a method proposed by Professor Bryan Caplan along with estimates of lockdown benefits based on the econometric evidence, I calculate a number of cost/benefit ratios of lockdowns in terms of life-years saved. Using a mid-point estimate for costs and benefits, the reasonable estimate for Canada is a cost/benefit ratio of 141. It is possible that lockdown will go down as one of the greatest peacetime policy failures in modern history.[154]

5.4.2 *Martin Lally's CBA for New Zealand*

In New Zealand, Professors Michael Baker[155] and Nick Wilson of Otago University recommended lockdown on 19 March 2020 thus: "New Zealand should consider a short pulse (a few weeks) of intense social distancing, including bringing forward the school holidays and temporary closures of most businesses, social meeting places and public transport."[156] They added that "[t]he strongest evidence that containment works comes from the remarkable success of China in reversing a large outbreak" (*ibid*).

Subsequently, Martin Lally[157] conducted a CBA of New Zealand's lockdowns and concluded that "the nation-wide lockdown strategy was not warranted." He explains that he takes the "approach of assessing the savings in quality adjusted life years and comparing them to a standard benchmark figure" to ensure "that all quality adjusted life years saved by various health interventions are treated equally,

---

[154] Allen, Douglas W. (2021). "Covid-19 Lockdown Cost/Benefits: A Critical Assessment of the Literature," in *International Journal of the Economics of Business*, 21 September 2021, https://www.tandfonline.com/doi/abs/10.1080/13571516.2021.1976051.

[155] This person bears no relation to my eponymous co-author on *The Great Covid Panic*.

[156] University of Otago (2020). Why New Zealand needs to continue decisive action to contain coronavirus, 20 March 2020, https://bit.ly/3yUqJ9k.

[157] Lally, Martin (2021). "The Costs and Benefits of Covid-19 Lockdowns in New Zealand," in *medRxiv*, 27 July 2021, https://doi.org/10.1101/2021.07.15.21260606.

which accords with the ethical principle of equity across people." He finds that "a Cost per Quality Adjusted Life Year saved by locking down in March 2020" is "at least 13 times the generally employed threshold figure of $62,000 for health interventions in New Zealand." If one uses Lally's mid-range estimate for the value of a healthy life year, rather than the high-end estimate he uses in his paper, the costs of lockdowns in New Zealand were around 25 times any benefits.[158]

In other words, Lally finds that the cost to society of saving quality-adjusted COVID lives via lockdowns, even assuming that these lives did actually get saved by lockdowns, is far higher than that of other life-saving public health policies that could have been adopted instead.

5.4.3 *Selected other papers*

Many other studies have been produced that in some fashion weigh the likely harms and benefits of COVID lockdown policies. A selected few are outlined below for illustrative purposes.

- On 5 May 2020, Peter Castleden and Nick Hudson of PANDA published a draft cost-benefit analysis of lockdowns in South Africa.[159] A 10 May 2020 version[160] estimates that lockdowns may prevent up to 445,901 years of lost life, while lockdowns could cost at least 14 million years of lost life. Comparing the highest benefit from lockdowns with expected harms, the CBA estimated that costs exceed benefits by at least 30 times.[161]

- In May 2020, the Copenhagen Consensus Center reported the outcomes of its cost-benefit analysis of moderate social distancing in response to the COVID-19 pandemic in Ghana. The analysis recognised many costs of restrictions, including the loss of life

---

[158] http://youtu.be/dp_4HBRm-8c.

[159] Cowen, Tyler (2020). "Should South Africa lock down?" in Marginal Revolution blog, 7 May 2020, https://bit.ly/3Gd602k.

[160] Pandemics – Data and Analytics (PANDA) (2020). "Quantifying Years of Lost Life in South Africa Due to COVID-19," 11 May 2020, https://bit.ly/3PuNJBA.

[161] Business Live (2020). "EXCLUSIVE: Lockdown disaster dwarfs Covid-19, say SA actuaries," 5 May 2020, https://bit.ly/3wCw97k.

and livelihoods they would entail of people far younger than the average COVID victim, and the broad conclusion was that "a policy of moderate movement and livelihood restrictions will leave Ghana much worse off."[162]

- The UK Department of Health and Social Care, Office for National Statistics, Government Actuary's Department and Home Office on 15 July 2020 published a report using the currency of Quality-Adjusted Life Years (QALYs) and stating that "when morbidity is taken into account, the estimates for the health impacts from a lockdown and lockdown induced recession are greater in terms of QALYs than the direct COVID-19 deaths."[163]

- A July 2020 paper by Chaudhry et al in *EClinical Medicine* found that government actions such as border closures, full lockdowns, and a high rate of COVID-19 testing have not been found to be associated with statistically significant reductions in the number of COVID critical cases or overall mortality.[164]

- On 18 September 2020 a paper was released by Ben W. Mol and Jonathan Karnon[165] comparing Sweden to Denmark. In the authors' words, "[c]omparisons of public health interventions for COVID-19 should take into account life years saved and not only lost lives. Strict lockdown costs more than US$130,000 per life year saved. As our all our assumptions were in favour of strict lockdown, a flexible social distancing policy in response to COVID-19 is defensible."

---

[162] Copenhagen Consensus Centre (2020). *A rapid cost-benefit analysis of moderate social distancing in response to the COVID-19 pandemic in Ghana*, 20 May 2020, https://bit.ly/3MzZ818.

[163] Department of Health and Social Care, Office for National Statistics, Government Actuary's Department and Home Office (2020). Direct and Indirect Impacts of COVID-19 on Excess Deaths and Morbidity: Executive Summary, 15 July 2020, https://bit.ly/3MGfFAz.

[164] "A country-level analysis measuring the impact of government actions, country preparedness and socioeconomic factors on COVID-19 mortality and related health outcomes," https://www.thelancet.com/journals/eclinm/article/PIIS2589-5370(20)30208-X/fulltext.

[165] Ben W. Mol and Jonathan Karnon (2020). "Strict lockdown versus flexible social distance strategy for COVID-19 disease: a cost-effectiveness analysis," in *medRxiv*, https://doi.org/10.1101/2020.09.14.20194605.

- On 21 October 2020 an expert in infectious disease and critical care, Dr Ari Joffe of the Stollery Children's Hospital and the University of Alberta, was reported to have found that the cost of lockdowns in Canada was at least 10 times higher than the benefit in terms of population health and well-being. His analysis, which accounts for numerous variables such as economic recession, social isolation and impacts on life expectancy, education, and other health-care priorities – both in Canada and worldwide – was published in February 2021.[166]

- Prof John Gibson of New Zealand of the University of Waikato produced the following three papers in 2020:

  o "Hard, not early: Putting the New Zealand Covid-19 response in context," *New Zealand Economic Papers.*[167]

  o "Government mandated lockdowns do not reduce Covid-19 deaths: Implications for evaluating the stringent New Zealand response," *New Zealand Economic Papers.*[168]

  o "Direct and indirect effects of Covid-19 on life expectancy and poverty in Indonesia," *Bulletin of Indonesian Economic Studies.*[169]

In a video summarising these papers,[170] Dr Gibson estimated that 10,000 times as many years of life will likely be lost by lockdowns in Indonesia relative to the life-years lost due to COVID deaths:

---

[166] Staples, David (2020). "Lockdowns will cause 10 times more harm to human health than COVID-19 itself, says infectious disease expert," in Edmonton Journal, 21 October 2020, https://archive.ph/XyPmt; Joffe, Ari R. (2021). "COVID-19: Rethinking the Lockdown Groupthink," in *Frontiers in Public Health*, 26 February 2021, https://www.frontiersin.org/articles/10.3389/fpubh.2021.625778/full.

[167] https://www.tandfonline.com/doi/full/10.1080/00779954.2020.1842796, Gibson, John (2020), "Hard, not early: putting the New Zealand Covid-19 response in context," in *New Zealand Economic Papers*.

[168] Gibson, John (2020). "Government mandated lockdowns do not reduce Covid-19 deaths: implications for evaluating the stringent New Zealand response," *New Zealand Economic Papers*, https://www.tandfonline.com/doi/full/10.1080/00779954.2020.1844786.

[169] Gibson, John (2020). "Direct and Indirect Effects of Covid-19 On Life Expectancy and Poverty in Indonesia," in *Bulletin of Indonesian Economic Studies*, https://www.tandfonline.com/doi/full/10.1080/00074918.2020.1847244.

[170] http://youtu.be/O2JOg4ki_so.

"the indirect effects on life expectancy, which operate through lower future income, exceed the direct effects of Covid-19-related deaths by at least five orders of magnitude." This figure is high because of the expectation that 20 to 25 million people are going to enter poverty due to the COVID lockdowns. In comparison, at minute 25 in his video, Prof Gibson suggests that with a 7% expected lower GDP due to lockdowns, New Zealanders would have a 1.2 percent lower life expectancy, equivalent to one year of lost life. That is more than 12 times larger than the direct harm to human well-being via expected COVID deaths, even if New Zealand had followed "relaxed" policies like Sweden.

- On 1 March 2021 Dr Sebastian Rushworth, a medical doctor in Sweden, opined that "the number of years of life lost to lockdown is many times greater than the number of years of life lost to covid-19."[171]

- On 22 March 2021, an op-ed by John Tierney in the *New York Post* claimed that lockdowns killed people on net.[172] In his words:

  More than two dozen studies have challenged the effectiveness of lockdowns, showing that closing businesses and schools does little or nothing to reduce infections and deaths from the virus.

  If a corporation behaved this way, continuing knowingly to sell an unproven drug or medical treatment with fatal side effects, its executives would be facing lawsuits, bankruptcy and criminal charges. But the lockdown proponents are recklessly staying the course, still insisting that lockdowns work.

  The burden of proof rests with those imposing such a dangerous policy, and they haven't met it. There is still no proof that lockdowns save any lives – let alone enough to compensate for the lives they end.

---

[171] Rushworth, Sebastian (2021). "Lockdowns have killed millions," 1 March 2021, https://bit.ly/3GdrThY.

[172] Tierney, John (2021). "The data shows lockdowns end more lives than they save," in *New York Post*, 22 March 2021, https://bit.ly/3G9gYpi.

Other CBAs have been produced by Andy Ryan in Ireland[173] and Christian Krekel, Richard Layard, and others[174] in the UK.

The list above does not include some CBAs, such as that penned by Richard Holden and Bruce Preston in *The Conversation*,[175] which make elementary errors in their approach and therefore would not survive robust scientific review or an independent peer review.

---

[173] Ryan, A. (2021). "A Cost–Benefit Analysis of the COVID-19 Lockdown in Ireland," 10.2139/ssrn.3872861, 16 June 2021, https://papers.ssrn.com/sol3/papers.cfm?abstract_id=3872861.

[174] Frijters, P., Clark, A.E., Krekel, C., & Layard, R. (2020). "A happy choice: Wellbeing as the goal of government," in *Behavioural Public Policy*, 4(2), 126-165. 10.1017/bpp.2019.39, https://bit.ly/38HRT8U.

[175] Frijters, Paul (2020). "The corona cost-benefit analyses of Richard Holden, Bruce Preston and Neil Bailey: ooops!" in *Club Troppo*, 18 May 2020, https://bit.ly/3wBvDX6.

PART II

COST-BENEFIT ANALYSIS OF AUSTRALIA'S LOCKDOWNS

6. Methodological issues and definitions

In this chapter I make a few observations on methodological issues. My approach to conducting a cost-benefit analysis of the Australian COVID lockdowns, using human well-being as a currency in which to count up the costs and benefits of a policy, is reasonably new, requiring the definition of some terms and a brief defence of the approach.

First, no cost-benefit analysis of any flavour is perfect. While it might be closest to the economists' ideal of weighing up "total surplus" created or destroyed by a policy, a utilitarian CBA (e.g., one requiring interpersonal "utility" comparisons) is theoretically impossible due to the inability to measure "utility." Conventional CBAs use the far more measurable currency of dollars, and sometimes when required and possible, Quality-Adjusted Life Years (QALYs). QALYs are translated as needed into dollars using an exchange rate drawn from society's observed willingness to pay for QALYs, which itself is deduced from a country's health expenditure decisions on behalf of its people. CBAs of this type are far from perfect – neither dollars nor QALYs are well-suited to capturing much of what makes like worth living, such as relationships, mental health, and social respect – but governments around the world use them because there is no more defensible way than a CBA to make judgments about policies that have myriad effects in different areas. Such judgements would otherwise become purely subjective and dependent on the whims of a single policy maker or group, potentially with inadequate accounting for the expected benefits and harms to all of society from different policy options. In sum, without the discipline of a transparent CBA to support our major policies, Australia's policy decision-making process would be far worse, with potentially catastrophic consequences for policy selection. Sadly, we have seen what this can lead to during the COVID era.

As they are in principle free of the influence of the emotions and whims of a single individual, CBAs are particularly well-suited to guiding decisions during times of high fear. Basic CBAs can be crafted quickly if needed. A whiteboard list of cost and benefits, created collectively and classified by informed people as "high," "medium" or "low," is often sufficient to provide a starting point for discussion. Even then however, representation of diverse sections of society that could be helped or harmed by a policy is crucial for producing a CBA that fulfills its potential to guide policymaking in an objective manner. Economics is the sole profession that aims to understand the holistic, "general equilibrium" results on society as a whole of any policy action, and also the discipline that most strongly promotes the consideration of the trade-offs and opportunity costs inherent in any action. It is thus no surprise that economists are the professionals in governments around the world who are usually tasked with generating CBAs.

Issues broader than crafting CBAs arise when considering Australia's COVID policies, such as whether lockdowns – which end up harming person X (say, a child or young person) in order to allegedly save person Y (say, an elderly person at risk from COVID) – are even morally acceptable or permissible under the law. A full consideration of such philosophical and legal questions is beyond the scope of this report.

6.1 Netting out the effect of lockdowns, over and above the counterfactual

If the Australian government had followed its pre-March 2020 official pandemic management plans, we would have seen the emergence of COVID followed by recommendations for voluntary social distancing and handwashing, and a very few mandatory public health orders. It is this world of "doing what we had planned to do" that will constitute the counterfactual case to which the policy Australia actually selected will be compared.

Even under the counterfactual, the following effects are likely:

- Because of the fear of disease, some people would reduce their supply of labour and interactions with others (e.g., avoiding restaurants or crowded places). This would affect the economy.
- Some people might choose to wear masks, and might experience some mental stress.
- Some people might choose to avoid hospitals, due to the fear of catching covid.

Such harms could have been reduced by calming messages from the government – messages that Australian governments conspicuously did not provide after mid-March 2020 – but arguably they would not have been avoided entirely. Because the above choices would have been based on individual risk levels,[176] the harms from these choices would be expected to be lower than the overall social benefit of the voluntary measures – but these harms would still have happened and should not be attributed to lockdowns.

Methodologically, it is challenging to separate the lockdown harms from harms that would have occurred in the counterfactual case. Some options for netting out the harms of a counterfactual policy are as follows:

- We could compare the magnitude and distribution of harms in Australia to those in Sweden, or in other countries or regions that did not impose lockdown policies.
- We could compare the harms in Australia with the harms Australia experienced during previous respiratory pandemics when lockdowns were not applied.
- We could regress various harm measures on the level of policy stringency using data from across regions or countries, and use the predicted values of harms based on the estimation results from

---

[176] The assumption here is that the individual person takes personal precautions that are roughly proportionate to his actual level of risk. This preservation of rationality is a normal assumption in CBAs, but it is threatened by a panic such as the one that gripped the world in March 2020. This is one reason why calm, sane government messaging, urging people to take those precautions that actually made sense given their situations, is a feature of the counterfactual policy scenario.

levels of stringency that match what the Australian counterfactual case would have looked like. Lally[177] used such an approach to gauge the extent to which the degree of policy stringency affects COVID deaths. A similar approach could potentially be used to determine if higher stringency causes other harms.

Unfortunately, the detailed data on harms that would be required for these analyses is not readily available. For most categories of harm, I therefore take a more pragmatic approach of using evidence-based but ballpark estimates of the likely amount of harm that would have occurred in the counterfactual case.

6.2 Assessing human welfare and quality of life

Australian governments tend to use discounted present values of both the harms and the benefits of policy alternatives, and where that is not practical, multi-criteria analysis is often applied. Such approaches, illustratively detailed in the *Victorian Guide to Regulation*, are consistent with the approach taken in the Green Book of the UK Treasury.[178]

Two related currencies can be used to gauge the implicit maximand of "human welfare" that can be harmed or helped via policy: the QALY and the WELLBY.

6.2.1 *Valuing life "equally"*

Some people, like Devi Sridhar, have expressed the view that all lives should be valued equally.[179] According to this view, a society must assign the same value to the life of a 5-year-old child as to the life of a person aged 105 when deciding how to spend scarce taxpayer dollars.

---

[177] Lally, Martin (2021). "The Costs and Benefits of Covid-19 Lockdowns in New Zealand," in *medRxiv*, 27 July 2021, https://doi.org/10.1101/2021.07.15.21260606.

[178] The UK Government (2020). The Green Book and accompanying guidance and documents, https://bit.ly/3wM8Syu.

[179] E.g., see Holden, Richard et al (2020). "'QALY' quality of life pandemic argument is intellectual malpractice," in *Sydney Morning Herald*, 24 September 2020, https://bit.ly/3MDL8U1.

This approach is not how public policy is generally made, and arguably would also fail on ethical grounds. Instead, what is conventionally done is to value a healthy human life-year equally across people, no matter to whom it accrues.

6.2.2 Assessing the quality of health: Quality-Adjusted Life-Years (QALYs)

Given scarce resources and time, society must, tragically, prioritise. In ethically fraught situations like battlefield triage, or when decisions are made about who should get scarce organs or which drugs should be included in the Pharmaceutical Benefits Scheme, policymakers recognise that saving a 20-year-old means saving more human welfare, in expectation, than saving an 80-year-old. This recognition is embodied in the concept of both QALYs and WELLBYs. The use of the QALY is cited in official Australian government documents as a standard approach to value non-fatal health outcomes.[180]

COVID deaths that may have been prevented via wholesale lockdowns are mainly of people over 70 years of age. As at 20 April 2022, the median age of those who die with COVID was 83,[181] virtually identical to the life expectancy of the average Australian born today. The average age of those who die with COVID will be higher still, given how few young people die with COVID. It would be unethical to ignore these realities when assessing the costs and benefits of any policy adopted in the fight against COVID.

The standard QALY currency using which health policy is typically evaluated is best regarded as a health QALY, although some authors have added aspheres of life beyond health to propose a broader "well-being QALY."[182] I will use the standard QALY in this report.

---

[180] An undated document by the Australian Institute of Health and Welfare (https://bit.ly/39H3ftM) discusses disability weights, QALY weights, health state valuations, health state preferences and health state utilities.

[181] Department of Health, Australian Government (2022). Coronavirus (COVID-19) at a glance – 20 April 2022, https://archive.ph/vqlfb.

[182] E.g., Cookson, R., Skarda, I., Cotton-Barratt, O., Adler, M., Asaria, M., & Ord, T. (2021). "Quality adjusted life years based on health and consumption: A summary well-being measure for cross-sectoral economic evaluation," in *Health economics*, 30(1), 70-85, https://doi.org/10.1002/hec.4177.

6.2.3 *Assessing life satisfaction: Wellbeing Years (WELLBYs)*

For assessing the harms of highly disruptive interventions like lock-downs, we need a way to take psychological and social factors into account. Such factors include mental health costs, loneliness, and social isolation; the cost of reduced immunity while we are sitting at home instead of being outside and enjoying time with friends; stress caused by unemployment and other effects on jobs; effects on people's savings; the stress of masking; effects on social and political stability; the pain of missing friends and family; the inability to make long-term plans; and the theft of freedom and privacy. There are also costs paid later because of lockdowns implemented today, such as those created by huge increases in government debt and the longer-run health damage of delaying treatment for non-COVID illnesses.

If such costs count, which they should in a balanced CBA just as much as should the costs of COVID disease, including longer-run impacts in both cases, then we need a common currency in which to measure both these costs and the costs of COVID-related deaths and suffering. That currency can in principle be quality-adjusted life-years, statistical lives, or a more direct measure of well-being. Which to choose?

While QALYs are commonly used to measure welfare gains when making decisions about the allocation of scarce resources, QALYs do not count the importance of many life dimensions that lockdowns directly damage. QALYs do not count loneliness, mental health suffering, loss of dignity or loss of joy. Statistical lives are a useful currency in cases where the average person's risk of dying is the key policy target, but this does not fit the COVID lockdown setting both because the average person is not at serious risk of dying from COVID, and because lockdowns involve damage to the quality of life that the statistical lives currency is not designed to accommodate.

Such costs are better amenable to quantification via the recently developed currency of well-being life-years, or WELLBYs.[183] Some background information about WELLBYs is provided below for readers unfamiliar with this relatively new currency.

A brief background on WELLBYs

The WELLBY method expands the QALY concept to the whole of the life experience, rather than focussing narrowly on health. The WELLBY captures the sorts of harms to human well-being that are difficult to capture in traditional ways, such as lost relationships, heightened anxiety, or lost motivation. WELLBYs have the advantage that they can be translated to QALYs, and thereby to dollars.

The WELLBY method was first proposed by Paul Frijters et al in 2019. These authors write:

> A natural name for the well-being experienced over one year is a Well-Being-Year (or WELLBY). What we want to maximise, across people in all present and future generations, is their number of future WELLBYs - with one qualification. Things that happen in the future are increasingly uncertain the further we look, and we, therefore, apply a "pure time discount rate," δ

According to Frijters et al.:

> While there is a considerable amount of research suggesting that subjective wellbeing scores do reflect underlying well-being (and in a way that is at least partly comparable across individuals), the question of which is the best measure remains largely open ... The front-runner at the moment remains life-satisfaction, generically measured by the first question in the UK's Office of National Statistics wellbeing module: "Overall, how satisfied are you with your life nowadays" where a 0 is "not at all" and a 10 is "completely"... Life Satisfaction is thus, like QALYs, not a perfect measure and one would like to see a process via which challengers can emerge so as to take the place of the 'current best measure'.[184]

---

[183] Frijters, Paul et al (2019). A Happy Choice: Wellbeing as the Goal of Government. Centre for Economic Performance, Discussion Paper 1658, https://bit.ly/3LF4pmG.
[184] *Ibid.* Also see the published version of this working paper, Frijters, Paul et al (2020), "A happy choice: Wellbeing as the goal of government," Behavioural Public Policy, 4(2), 126-165. doi:10.1017/bpp.2019.39

Frijters et al note the following in *The Great Covid Panic*:

> One WELLBY is defined as a one-point increment on this answer scale, lasting for one year, for one person. As a rule of thumb, a healthy person living in the UK answers around an 8 to this overall life satisfaction question, while a level of 2 is reported to be as bad as no longer living at all. This means that a "healthy year of life" in the UK is worth 6 WELLBYs more than a life not worth living. An intuitive and "relatable" measure of human wellbeing, the WELLBY is strongly affected by mental health, social relations, the environment, and basically anything that makes life enjoyable and worthwhile. It is now used by the UK government and many others as the basis of judging the quality of the life someone is leading.

In practical terms, the following excerpt outlines how the measure of life satisfaction can be used to gauge the impact of various aspects of a person's condition or surroundings on the quality of his or her life:

> [L]ife-satisfaction is regressed upon log household income per head, years of education, whether or not unemployed, number of criminal convictions (times minus one), whether partnered, number of physical health conditions, and whether diagnosed as suffering from a depression or anxiety disorder. Prior to running this regression, the outcome and covariates are standardised with means of zero and standard deviations of one. The square of each coefficient measures the fraction of the explained variance of life-satisfaction that is independently captured by the variable in question. [185]

An advantage of a WELLBY-based approach is that it can stand alone or be added to a conventional CBA:

> [w]ellbeing analysis could simply be added to existing cost-benefit analyses by adopting a willingness-to-pay number for the value of a WELLBY.[186]

---

[185] *Ibid.*

[186] Frijters, Paul and Krekel, Christian (2021). *A Handbook for Wellbeing Policy-Making.* Oxford: Oxford University Press, page xvii.

Use of the WELLBY method in government analyses

While promising, the WELLBY is not yet used widely in government analyses. Frijters et al recommend that:

> the bureaucracy should adopt a current metric for wellbeing, i.e. life satisfaction, until a better one comes along. … [it] assumes … that happiness is measurable on a cardinal scale (like temperature) and that levels of happiness can be compared between one person and another.[187]

Further,

> for wellbeing to become the goal of government, it is necessary to systematically integrate a commonly agreed-upon small set of core wellbeing indicators – the principal being life satisfaction – in surveys regularly conducted by national statistical agencies. Following recommendations by Dolan et al (2011, 2012), the Office for National Statistics (ONS) in the UK has taken a lead role in measurement: starting in 2011, the agency has included (at least) four wellbeing indicators, covering evaluative, experiential, and eudemonic dimensions of wellbeing, in all of its surveys. [188]

The inclusion of an appendix on well-being cost-effectiveness analysis in the UK Treasury's Green Book is a signal of the traction and potential of the WELLBY within government policy-making circles.[189]

Relationship between WELLBYs and QALYs

The standard literature on WELLBYs considers that a healthy life year is worth 6 WELLBYs experienced by one person for one year, meaning that an extra WELLBY's worth of life is equivalent to one-sixth of a QALY's worth of life.

This equivalence is not set in stone. Cookson et al note: "If life satisfaction is measured on a ten-point scale, and if 2 is considered

---

[187] Frijters, Paul et al (2019). A Happy Choice: Wellbeing as the Goal of Government. Centre for Economic Performance, Discussion Paper 1658, https://bit.ly/3LF4pmG.
[188] *Ibid.*
[189] *Ibid.*

to represent a life barely worth living while 10 is a fully satisfactory life, then one WELLBY is approximately one eighth of a well-being QALY."[190]

I will use the standard exchange rate of 6 WELLBYs per QALY in this report when considering losses due to the shortening of lives. However, gaining an additional QALY via the quality-adjustment portion of the QALY measure (meaning due to improved health, not to higher longevity – or in colloquial shorthand, adding life to one's years rather than years to one's life) is only worth a gain of about 2.5 WELLBYs, because physical health is only one of the factors important for a satisfied life.

Limitations of the method used in this CBA

Many questions remain regarding the WELLBY method that also arise with traditional cost-benefit analysis. Among others, these include how to aggregate happiness across people or across time (including what discount rate is appropriate), and how to value the length of life and the birth rate in and of themselves.[191] Further consideration of such questions is beyond the scope of this paper.

6.3 The "precautionary principle" rejects CBA and good policymaking

The precautionary principle has been extensively invoked during the 2020 pandemic to justify extreme policies. For example, the following is contained in paragraph 20 of a letter sent on 15 March 2020 from the Chief Health Officer of Victoria, tabled in the Victorian Parliament, advising the Minister to declare a State of Emergency:

> In formulating advice, it is based upon the best available evidence, however I note that the lack of full scientific certainty should not be used as a reason for postponing measures to

---

[190] Cookson, R., Skarda, I., Cotton-Barratt, O., Adler, M., Asaria, M., & Ord, T. (2021). "Quality adjusted life years based on health and consumption: A summary wellbeing measure for cross-sectoral economic evaluation," in *Health economics*, 30(1), pp. 70-85, https://doi.org/10.1002/hec.4177.

[191] Frijters, Paul et al (2019). A Happy Choice: Wellbeing as the Goal of Government. Centre for Economic Performance, Discussion Paper 1658, https://bit.ly/3LF4pmG.

prevent or control the public health risk (section 6 of the Act).[192]

Section 6 of the Victorian *Public Health and Wellbeing Act 2008* provides the following working definition of the precautionary principle: "Precautionary principle: If a public health risk poses a serious threat, lack of full scientific certainty should not be used as a reason for postponing measures to prevent or control the public health risk."

The precautionary principle as stated above enables a decision-maker to evade assessing a policy's proportionality and absolves the government of the responsibility to provide a reasoned argument supporting policy efficacy, depending on the interpretation of a single word: "serious." Lockdown policies applied early in 2020 on the grounds of the precautionary principle were not challenged on the basis that lockdowns had been rejected in the past by scientists. They were not challenged on the basis that lockdowns had not been identified as a viable policy option in Victoria's pandemic plan for a threat like COVID. The precautionary principle effectively empowered the Chief Health Officer, advising the government of a sufficiently panicked people, to recommend an extreme measure as a "remedy" to that panic. The fact that the extreme policy measure was wholly unproven as a remedy for COVID was of no consequence because the threat was perceived by those operating in panic mode as "serious."

6.3.1 *Precaution against causing harm from lockdowns was not taken*

The Hippocratic Oath as commonly quoted today – "First, do no harm" – is perhaps the most famous precautionary principle. Instead of advocating unproven intervention "just in case," however, it demands the opposite kind of precaution: to not intervene when doing so may cause harm. The principle of "First, do no harm" could not be used to defend the government's attempt, with lockdowns, to avert

---

[192] Chief Health Officer Advice to Minister for Health. Victoria on 15 March 2020: Advice relating to Declaration of State of Emergency, tabled in the Parliament of Victoria, https://bit.ly/3Pyp3qQ.

COST-BENEFIT ANALYSIS OF AUSTRALIA'S LOCKDOWNS

a disease in advance by imposing an intervention with unproven efficacy that is known to cause harm.

To have been used in a meaningful way, the precautionary principle should have been applied not just to the threat of COVID, but also to the proposed lockdown policies themselves. Had that balanced consideration occurred, lockdowns would not have passed the test of precaution.

John Lee, former clinical professor of pathology at Hull York Medical School, made the following comments in the documentary entitled *UK Unlocked* about the misuse of the precautionary principle:[193]

> As a doctor one of the overriding medical principles is the Hippocratic principle, … first do no harm. You should be sure that what you're doing to them is going to cause a better outcome for that patient than doing nothing at all. … Yet it was one of the first casualties of the response to covid because the government decided to prescribe a treatment for the entire country with no risk-benefit analysis of that treatment whatsoever …

> One of the hidden aspects of this epidemic and its management it seems to me is the way that it is being driven by something called the precautionary principle and this is something that isn't widely understood amongst the general public … But it has become embedded in the political management of diseases and other health scares and the precautionary principle basically says that if there seems to be a potential harm to human health you shouldn't wait until all the scientific data is in demonstrating that harm to health before you take action to prevent the harms. But, of course, if you don't know scientifically that harms are really being caused in a certain way or by a certain mechanism, then it is actually a dangerous principle because it encourages politicians and public health doctors to take widespread intrusive actions on the basis of something that may not be true and without properly assessing the effects of those very actions themselves.

---

[193] http://youtu.be/btWfAXQ8wYg.

In fact, this last year what we've seen is the fruition of that principle on a huge scale. One of the ways in which the precautionary principle has exaggerated the response to covid is because it is based on worst case scenario planning. So, when SAGE, the Specialist Advisory Group on Emergencies, is asked to give the government answers to their questions they're asked to explain what the worst case scenario would be. But, of course, worst case scenario planning isn't a way that we ever normally live our lives. If we worked on the worst-case scenario, we'd never drive a car, we'd never catch an airplane, we'd never eat, we'd never get out of bed. It is not that you shouldn't consider worst-case scenarios but they're just one of many scenarios that you should consider.

6.3.2 *Was limited intervention justified at the very early stage?*

Taking a charitable view of the potential impact of the government's actions, could international border closures (which, like domestic lockdowns, carry costs) have been justified in the early weeks after COVID's emergence, for the reason of allowing time for the health and aged care systems to prepare for the expected stress of incoming COVID cases? That was certainly the reasoning used prominently to justify such closures at the time. Yet even such a short period of border closures conflicts with pre-2020 expert advice.

A 2017 hypothetical cost-benefit analysis of border closures for New Zealand for a "severe" pandemic noted that: "A widespread view is that country border closures have a limited, if any, role in preventing the spread of infectious diseases. Indeed, the World Health Organization (WHO) advice is that even though unaffected countries may be able to delay the introduction of the infectious agent by imposing severe limits on international travel, border closure is unlikely to be able to prevent importation, and can have huge economic and personal costs."[194] Consistent with this widely held view, the WHO's October 2019 guidelines indicate that border closures are

---

[194]   Boyd, Matt et al (2017). "Protecting an island nation from extreme pandemic threats: Proof-of-concept around border closure as an intervention," in *PLoS One,* https://www.ncbi.nlm.nih.gov/pmc/articles/PMC5473559/.

"not recommended" since it found a "very low" quality of evidence in support of this approach.[195]

To arrive at its recommendation, the WHO shortlisted 11 studies.[196] One of these suggested that border restrictions could delay an epidemic by 2-3 weeks. However, all 11 of them were deemed to have "very low" evidence quality and many did not control for other "confounding factors" such as pre-existing immunity. WHO guidelines suggest that border controls should preferably be voluntary even if a nation considers them (see page 95 of the WHO report's Annexure: "as with internal travel restriction, border controls should be voluntarily applied as much as possible, and compulsory intervention should be involved as a last resort").

As pointed out by Donald Henderson, border closures could not control even smallpox.[197] The 2017 self-described "proof of concept" CBA for New Zealand border closures cited above, which included as the direct economic costs of border closures only the estimated foregone tourism revenue, suggested that "more detailed cost-benefit analysis of border closure in very severe pandemic situations for some island nations is probably warranted, as this course of action might sometimes be worthwhile from a societal perspective." However, the other substantial costs of lockdowns enumerated in this report that were not counted in the 2017 CBA for New Zealand, in addition to the review of pre-2020 scientific consensus provided earlier, imply that even for island nations, policies like border closures would fail a complete cost-benefit test except in extremely exceptional circumstances and when fighting a threat of a different nature to COVID.

Whether even any temporary international border closures in March 2020 would have passed an *ex ante* cost-benefit test also de-

---

[195] Page 18 of the WHO'S 2019 guidelines, Non-pharmaceutical public health measures for mitigating the risk and impact of epidemic and pandemic influenza: https://bit.ly/39JCmFw.

[196] Details of these 11 studies are found at page 93 in the Appendix to the main October 2019 guidelines, at https://bit.ly/3sQ1pxc.

[197] Quoted from Donald Henderson's comments from timestamp 32:35 on a panel at the 5 March 2010 conference on "The 2009 H1N1 experience: Policy implications for future infectious disease emergencies," at http://youtu.be/8rEV857R0LE.

pends on detailed information about the pre-COVID state of Australia's health and aged care services sectors and the speed at which life-saving preparations could have been implemented. Answering these questions is beyond the scope of this report.

Any justification for temporary border closures would likely have petered out sometime in April 2020, by which point not only was knowledge about the nature and risk of the virus abundantly available, but the accumulated costs of continued closures would have almost surely outweighed any potential benefit (which would be chiefly in terms of delaying infections and the symptoms and deaths they led to) of extending them.

6.4 Potential methodological questions regarding COVID cases and deaths

Two types of concerns plague our ability to interpret statistical reports about COVID: an over-emphasis on COVID cases, and potential over-counting of COVID deaths. I do not draw a specific conclusion about the size of each problem in the Australian case, but merely sketch why reported statistics on these quantities must be treated gingerly.

6.4.1 *Suffering and deaths should matter, not cases*

The media has focused heavily on COVID cases. The relevant variable for public policy design, however, is human suffering or death due to COVID (or, for that matter, due to other things). These outcomes of interest are facilitated by underlying lack of health in the vulnerable population, poor prophylaxis, negligent early treatment, and transmission of the virus to those who are at risk of serious symptoms or death from the disease. Case counts matter far less than the number of people who are actually sick in hospital or dying. Further, there are concerns about the reliability and validity of PCR tests used across Australia as the primary source of data on case counts. The number of reported cases in a region is also mechanically related to the number of tests administered in that region. In sum, case numbers indicate something very different to outcomes of policy interest. The following information taken from the DHS website illustrates this:

> As at 3 pm on 2 October 2021, a total of 109,315 cases of COVID-19 have been reported in Australia, including 1,321 deaths, and approximately 21,472 active cases. The median age of all cases is 31 years (range: 0 to 106 years). The median age of deaths is 84 years (range: 15 to 106 years).[198]

The stark difference in the median age for cases (31 years) and deaths (84 years) tells us that most of those infected were young, but that the disease was generally not lethal to them. Taken at face value, these statistics also imply that more that 80% of COVID infections (i.e., all but (21,472+1,321) of 109,315 cases) resulted in recovery, and that COVID is minimally lethal even amongst those who decide to get tested and return a positive test (resulting in death for only 1,321 out of 109,315 reported cases, i.e., with a case survival rate of nearly 99%)), but those facts are not emphasised. We also see nothing in the above "COVID status report" about the severity of illnesses (e.g., hospitalisations or ICU beds occupied because of COVID).

The costly mass-scale testing we witnessed during the COVID era is unlikely to have passed an *ex ante* cost-benefit test for reasons such as these, but a full analysis of this question is beyond the scope of this report.

6.4.2 *How to know that a death is due to COVID*

On 25 March 2020, the Australian Bureau of Statistics wrote that a death can be merely assumed to be from COVID:

> The new coronavirus strain (COVID-19) should be recorded on the medical cause of death certificate for ALL decedents where the disease caused, or is assumed to have caused, or contributed to death.[199]

[198] Department of Health, Australian Government. Coronavirus (COVID-19) at a glance – 2 October 2021. https://archive.ph/8277G.
[199] Australian Bureau of Statistics (2020). Guidance for Certifying Deaths due to COVID-19, updated on 25 March 2020, https://bit.ly/3GbnLin.

The Coroners Court in Western Australia has used the following guidance on counting COVID deaths:

> Where a person is known to have suffered typical symptoms of COVID-19, such as fevers, cough, or breathing difficulties, during a COVID-19 pandemic, but has not been formally tested or diagnosed, then it is reasonable to "assume" the death was related to COVID-19 and should be recorded on the death certificate.[200]

The University of Melbourne (CRVS technical guide: Correctly certifying deaths due to COVID–19: Guidance for physicians[201]) has issued guidance stating that "there are two distinct ICD-10 codes used for coding COVID-19 deaths – U07.1 (COVID-19, virus identified) and U07.2 (COVID-19, virus not identified)". It then notes that "[e]valuation studies have shown that medical certificates of cause of death are often of poor quality, even when the cause of death has been certified by a physician."

Is it normal practice to have a code for COVID deaths (U07.2) when the virus was not even identified on the person? It is unclear whether such a method is adopted for other diseases. Does this method allow deaths from other respiratory viruses to be categorised as COVID deaths, given the overlap in symptoms between COVID and "regular" colds and flu – thereby inflating COVID death counts?

Although this does not appear to be the case in Australia, in some countries an even more extreme reporting protocol was reported, wherein every death within 28 days of a positive PCR was considered to be a COVID death.[202] While the BMJ considered this issue on 10 February 2021,[203] more work is needed to understand the full

---

[200] Coroner's Court, Western Australia. COVID-19 Guide for Medical Practitioners. https://bit.ly/3sRqCY9.

[201] University of Melbourne. CRVS technical guide: Correctly certifying deaths due to COVID–19: Guidance for physicians, May 2020. https://bit.ly/3lwE6of.

[202] A UK government blog discusses this issue: UK Health Security Agency (2020). Behind the headlines: Counting COVID-19 deaths, 12 August 2020, https://bit.ly/3NziyDz; to be read along with "COVID-19 deaths within 28 days of a positive COVID-19 test and ONS methodology for COVID-19 reporting" – https://bit.ly/3MHWTca.

[203] Oliver, David (2021). "Mistruths and misunderstandings about covid-19 death numbers," in *BMJ*, 10 February 2021, https://www.bmj.com/content/372/bmj.n352.

scope and implications of this convention. Some commentators have reported that in some countries there were no time limits, meaning that any deceased person who had ever returned a positive PCR test would have been counted as a COVID death.[204] This flags not only the possibility of inflated COVID death counts in general, but potential problems in comparing data on COVID deaths across nations.

6.4.3 Deaths "with," not "from," COVID

Isolating a single cause of death has always been a dubious exercise, since at the end of life many people suffer from multiple interdependent medical problems. It has become an even more dubious exercise during COVID times.

It was reported on 30 March 2020 by then recently retired professor of pathology Dr John Lee of the UK that "Many UK health spokespersons have been careful to repeatedly say that the numbers quoted in the UK indicate death with the virus, not death due to the virus – this matters. When giving evidence in parliament a few days ago, Prof Neil Ferguson of Imperial College London said that he now expects fewer than 20,000 Covid-19 deaths in the UK but, importantly, two-thirds of these people would have died anyway."[205]

In Australia it was reported by La Trobe University on 9 September 2020 that "[t]here's been confusion … over whether reported death statistics reflect those who've died from COVID-19, or those who've died with the virus. Often it's hard for medical practitioners to determine which of these categories a death falls into."[206]

The pattern of vulnerability to severe disease across individuals suggests that the progression of a COVID infection is assisted by age and pre-existing co-morbidities. Pinning down exactly what "caused" a given death, whether or not COVID was present, can be likened to trying to pin down a simple reason for any complex phenomenon, from civil war to suicide.

---

[204] Tweet by plaforscience dated 16 September 2021, https://bit.ly/3wK7Kvj.

[205] Lee, John (2020). "How to understand – and report – figures for 'Covid deaths'," in *The Spectator*, 30 March 2020, https://bit.ly/3aiuDP5.

[206] Trabsky, Marc (2020). "'Died from' or 'died with' COVID-19?" Latrobe University. https://bit.ly/38JPsT5.

Prima facie, Sweden's reporting protocols appear to have had an in-built tendency to over-report COVID deaths:

> Sweden chose a model that might over-report COVID-19 deaths: they do not require a death certificate stating CO-VID-19 is the cause of death, but also count all people who die with the virus (including post-mortem testing and all residential aged care facility [RACF] deaths) as COVID-19 deaths by automatically matching the national death registry with test results. In principle, an asymptomatic young person stepping out of the testing booth and getting run over by a bus would count as a COVID-19 death.[207]

This may explain why, although Sweden reported 9,800 COVID deaths in 2020, its excess deaths that year were only around 3000, implying that reported COVID deaths were exaggerated by up to a factor of three.

In comparison, *The Economist* has suggested that some countries likely under-reported COVID deaths. It points out that "Britain, Spain, Italy, Belgium and Portugal have some of the highest national excess-mortality rates in the world." However, *The Economist*'s methodology does not adjust for any country-specific factors, nor does it net out non-COVID deaths or flag that these may have resulted from COVID management policies, not COVID itself. As a reason for the under-reporting of deaths suggested, the authors recognise that "the pandemic has made it harder for doctors to treat other conditions and discouraged people from going to hospital, which may have indirectly caused an increase in fatalities from diseases other than covid-19."[208]

Even in the UK, however, there is some evidence of over-reporting, as illustrated by this newspaper article excerpt:[209]

---

[207] Herb, Horst (2020), "Was the Swedish approach to COVID-19 really a mistake?" in *NewsGP*, a blog of the Royal Australian College of General Practitioners, https://bit.ly/39KyTXa.
[208] *The Economist* (2020). Tracking covid-19 excess deaths across countries, https://bit.ly/3G9nVXq.
[209] Gilbody-Dickerson, Claire (2021). "Grieving families demand answers after deaths 'wrongly attributed to Covid,'" in *Mirror*, 27 February 2021, https://bit.ly/3lBQ0gy.

> Grieving families are calling for an inquiry into how deaths have been recorded during the pandemic amid claims their loved ones did not die of Covid.
>
> Dozens of families are said to have raised concerns after Bel Mooney revealed that her father, 99, who suffered from dementia and chronic obstructive pulmonary disease, had his death recorded as coronavirus.
>
> Bel claimed her dad had passed three Covid-19 tests but was nonetheless registered as one of the 122,000 people who have died of the virus in the UK.
>
> She said when she sought an explanation for this, the care home doctor explained it was because there had been some Covid-related deaths on the same dementia floor.

There have also been some reports about changes to definitions relevant to counting deaths for COVID compared with counting deaths for similar diseases in the past, and some reports of changes midway through the COVID era about how COVID deaths are counted.[210]

In some countries, reporting COVID activity (cases, deaths, vaccines) may have been associated in some manner with financial incentives for hospitals, doctors, or nursing homes.[211] In the US for example, Professor Jay Bhattacharya of Stanford has spoken about "strong incentives to overreport [COVID deaths]."[212] Claims of this nature have been rejected by mainstream media in Australia.[213]

A full investigation of reporting protocols and possible financial incentives – including the technical comparisons of International Classification of Diseases (ICD) definitions and how these were used relative to what was done for similar respiratory viruses in the

---

[210] E.g., Smyth, Chris (2020). "Coronavirus: New method of counting slashes official death toll," in *The Times*. https://bit.ly/3PBfYPb.

[211] Evidence provided in a complaint by Sanjeev Sabhlok to the International Criminal Court (https://bit.ly/3yT7HAm) and at http://youtu.be/ga2FzSsOcpw.

[212] http://youtu.be/D6HFivRezzI.

[213] E.g., RMIT ABC Fact Check. "Why you shouldn't believe the rumours about nursing homes being paid for COVID-19 deaths," in *ABC News*, https://bit.ly/3LCXQRM.

past – that would be required to clarify such issues is beyond the scope of this report.

Overall, the precise number of deaths that would not have occurred but for COVID remains unclear, for a variety of interdependent reasons. Regardless, I use official figures in this report, but to the extent possible I prefer to use excess deaths as a more accurate measure of death due to COVID and/or due to our response to it. As epidemiologist Dr Raghib Ali notes:

> [L]ooking at just Covid-19 mortality doesn't give the full picture as different counties code deaths in different ways and so we need to look at excess mortality, which is the best comparative measure.[214]

---

[214] Ali, Raghib (2021). "Would an earlier lockdown really have saved tens of thousands of lives?" in *The Telegraph*, 21 March 2021, https://bit.ly/39HxoJq.

7. Illustrative cost-benefit analysis of UK lockdowns (from *The Great Covid Panic*)

In my 2021 book, *The Great Covid Panic* – referred to hereafter in this chapter as 'TGCP' – my co-authors and I outline a CBA of the UK's lockdowns. I summarise our analysis in this chapter in order to demonstrate the logic and method of such CBAs.

7.1 Benefits of UK lockdowns (as assessed in *The Great Covid Panic*)

7.1.1 *COVID deaths prevented*

To be conservative and favourable to the policies actually enacted, TGCP assumes that lockdowns were capable of stopping all expected COVID deaths in the UK. In TGCP we assume an upper bound of 3,000 per million COVID deaths prevented by lockdowns. Data from Worldometer as at 4 July 2022 suggest that the UK has had 2,630 COVID deaths per million to date.

In TGCP we argue that since the average COVID death in the UK has been of someone above 80 years of age and in poor health, often in a nursing home where those who enter have the equivalent of about one more healthy year of life left, it is reasonable to assume that the average COVID death takes away about three healthy years of human life. This is equivalent to 18 WELLBYs, since a healthy life year is worth 6 WELLBYs.

Therefore, the total WELLBY loss that lockdowns could possibly have saved the UK from experiencing (i.e., of 3,000 deaths per million prevented from dying from COVID) is 3000 x 6 x 3 = **54,000** WELLBYs *per million*.

Unlike the per-month costs that lockdowns create, enumerated in Table 7.1 below, this is a total benefit. As an update to what was known at the time of writing TGCP, the UK announced an end to all

COVID restrictions on 21 February 2022, meaning that the COVID deaths averted by lockdowns, whatever their number, have at this point all been averted.[215]

7.1.2 *Longer-term costs of COVID*

Longer-term costs of COVID include "long COVID" and the possibility of new viral strains emerging.

7.1.2.1 *Long COVID*

As the months wore on, worry emerged about 'long COVID', the phenomenon wherein some people who recovered from an acute bout of COVID infection had lingering health problems for months afterward. If these problems involve significant long-term human costs, then we should include them in our estimate of the potential WELLBY loss due directly to COVID.

A consortium of Swiss doctors,[216] organised during the pandemic to work quickly through the rapidly evolving scientific knowledge on COVID, noted that recovery from many viral infections can take a long time, so 'long COVID' was not unexpected or unusual. They noted that the percentage of COVID sufferers who still had symptoms after three months varied across studies from between 2% and 10% of patients, and that there was little evidence of permanent damage. My reading of the currently available research on this topic concurs with the view of these Swiss doctors, published in June 2021.

The most recent understanding is that nearly every COVID victim does totally recover, but in some cases it can take several months.[217] During the recovery period, life is a bit worse for long COVID sufferers but most are still able to socialise, meaning that their well-being is impaired relatively modestly. Compared to deaths and the other

---

[215] CBS News (2022). "British Prime Minister Boris Johnson announces end to all COVID restrictions in England, 21 February 2022," https://archive.ph/ADDs7.

[216] Swiss Policy Research. "Post-Acute Covid and Long Covid," updated January 2022, https://bit.ly/3MD1egB.

[217] Swiss Policy Research. "Post Covid Syndrome ("Long Covid")," updated August 2021, https://bit.ly/3yVGOeS.

costs enumerated in Table 7.1 (below), this means that the negative well-being effect of long COVID is relatively small – on the order of 1% to 5% of the WELLBY effects of 0.3% of the population dying of COVID.

7.1.2.2 *Uncertainties about new strains*

A bigger worry about the long-run direct costs of COVID is that COVID is not a single viral strain, but more like an evolving cloud of strains with new mutations emerging all the time, like the influenza virus. How can we approach quantifying the long-run costs of a seasonally recurring illness that is always somewhat novel and can to some extent resist previous vaccines – and are such longer-run costs plausibly prevented via lockdowns implemented now?

The notion of a 'fatality rate' applies to an identified strain or a small bandwidth of strains. By contrast, a recurring and perennially evolving group of viruses like seasonal flu or seasonal COVID is better thought of in terms of its effect on life expectancy: i.e., how many weeks or months does it cost people? That number is unknown at the time of writing, because it remains to be seen whether new COVID strains will evolve and circulate every year. However, this does not affect our consideration of the trade-offs inherent in lockdowns. The costs and benefits of trying to control a mutating virus that comes back every year in a slightly different form are more or less the aggregate of the costs and benefits of the series of actions targeted to the series of mutant strains. I therefore focus on the costs and benefits of the initial COVID lockdowns, acknowledging that a parallel analysis could be performed in relation to the actions taken to fight every strain.[218]

---

[218] A more comprehensive analysis would include not only the benefits of policies in terms of combatting each major variant, but also the impact of these policies on future variants. The endogeneity of variant progression would be recognised and accounted for. Among the factors to be considered by such a complex analysis would be: (a) the loss of society's immunity due to lockdowns; (b) a reduction in viral replication and hence mutation speed due to lockdowns; and (c) the likely direction of successful mutations, which in the case of respiratory viruses is largely towards enhanced contagion and reduced severity, although some exceptions may exist (USA Today. "Fact check: Yes, viruses can mutate to become more deadly," 14 July 2021, https://bit.ly/3Ly2Sih). This

7.2 Costs of UK lockdowns (assessed in *The Great Covid Panic*)

Table 7.1 (a reproduction of Table 5 from TGCP) displays our estimates of the costs per month of a UK-style lockdown, per million citizens, denominated in WELLBYs. Similar losses to those in Table 7.1 are found in many Western countries. These estimates indicate how much disruption lockdowns bring to the developed West and how many dimensions of our lives they affect.

Disrupted area	Loss in original units	Loss in WELLBYs
IVF services	30 IVF babies lost	14,400
Satisfaction with life	0.5 on a 0-10 scale	41,667
Future health problems	429 extra deaths	12,857
Government debt	US$514 million	51,400
Pollution	no effect	0
Suicide	?	0
Child education	20-30% time lost	5,714
Total		126,038

Table 7.1: Costs per Month of Lockdowns, per One Million Citizens, United Kingdom

An explanation of the line items in Table 7.1 is provided below.

7.2.1 *Line 1: IVF babies who were never born*

In a country like the UK, around 3% of births each year are the result of in-vitro fertilisation.[219] IVF services were halted during lockdowns according to the logic that IVF was a 'nonessential' service not worth the 'risk.' As a result, around 2,000 births per month of lockdown

would suggest that quicker viral mutation away from the initial strain (meaning, potentially, a higher amount of early transmission among those who are less vulnerable) may be optimal from the perspective of producing a less dangerous health threat as quickly as possible. Such an analysis is outside the scope of this paper, but at the very least it may be premature to judge whether any reduced transmission produced by lockdowns was a good thing or a bad thing in the long run.

[219] E.g., see Slater, Annabel (2021). "The Health of IVF Babies: What Do We Know? What Do We Need to Find Out?" in BioNews, 1 March 2021. https://bit.ly/3G9mYhL.

will not have happened that otherwise would have. Given the UK population of around 70 million, this translates to about 30 fewer IVF births per million citizens per month.

Those babies would have been expected on average to live in good health for around 80 years. One year of good health is worth about six WELLBYs. Therefore, the 30 lost IVF babies per month could each have expected to enjoy 480 WELLBYs in his or her life, meaning the UK lost **14,400 WELLBYs' worth of human well-being per month per million citizens** as a direct result of the policy-mandated disruption to IVF services in lockdowns.

7.2.2 *Line 2: Satisfaction with life*

The second type of cost listed in Table 7.1, under the heading 'Satisfaction with life', refers to the damage done to the well-being of the whole population during the period of lockdowns. We capture here the loss of happiness attributable to the disruptions, and all of the mental health problems caused by increased loneliness, physical abuse from domestic violence, and diminution of purpose. This item also captures the possibility that many people rather like lockdowns and feel quite comfortable locked away with their families: they impact the statistics by moderating the drop in life satisfaction. Yet, on net, we see a high loss of well-being, showing that the costs to the losers far outweigh the gains to the winners. We see evidence of these net well-being costs in other statistics such as the percentage of the population with depression and anxiety, which rose from around 16% to 25% in this period in the UK, a scale of impact also seen in other countries.[220]

We also know from many studies that this well-being loss increased as lockdowns dragged on and people became more de-

---

[220] Kathryn E. Mansfield et al (2021). "Indirect acute effects of the COVID-19 pandemic on physical and mental health in the UK: a population-based study," in *The Lancet*, Volume 3, Issue 4, E217-E230, 1 April 2021 (published online on February 18, 2021), https://doi.org/10.1016/S2589-7500(21)00017-0.

pressed and lonely.[221] The average effect of lockdowns in the UK until March 2021 was around 0.5 of a WELLBY,[222] an effect also found for other places like Australia which had well-defined lockdown periods in particular regions.[223] A drop of 0.5 WELLBYs (a yearly measure) translates to a drop of 0.5/12 per month per person, or **41,667 WELLBYs per month per million UK citizens.** This means that in about three weeks of lockdown, the well-being lost due to loneliness and other mental health effects is equivalent to that lost from all COVID deaths that occurred in the UK through June 2021.

7.2.3 *Line 3: Future health problems*

Moving to the third item in Table 7.1, our estimate of deaths from future health problems caused by disruption to health services comes directly from a UK government report of December 2020.[224] This report claimed that 100,000 Britons would die in the future because of health-service disruption in the six months after March 2020. If we conservatively estimate that each of those deaths – for example, a preventable cancer death attributable to reduced cancer screening – causes the loss of five years of healthy human life, then the total cost of health-service disruptions equates to **12,857 WELLBYs lost per million citizens per month** of lockdown.

---

[221] *The Conversation* discusses a recent meta-analysis of 33 studies (Karantzas, Gery (2022). "Lockdowns doubled your risk of mental health symptoms," https://bit.ly/3LCjfdR) – see https://www.sciencedirect.com/science/article/pii/S2352250X22000252, where the study is available. It states that "Social restrictions were significantly associated with increased mental health symptoms overall, including depression, stress and loneliness, but not anxiety." In brief: "We found that overall, social restrictions doubled people's odds of experiencing mental health symptoms."

[222] See, for example, Figure 2 in Office for National Statistics (2021), "Data collection changes due to the pandemic and their impact on estimating personal well-being," https://bit.ly/3wDFH27.

[223] Biddle, N., et al (2020). "Hardship, distress, and resilience: The initial impacts of COVID-19 in Australia," ANU Centre for Social Research and Methods, 7 May 2020, https://apo.org.au/node/303652.

[224] DHSC/ONS/GAD/HO: "Direct and indirect impacts of COVID-19 on excess deaths and morbidity – December 2020 update, 17 December 2020," 29 January 2021, https://bit.ly/3wLwgMz (mainly items C1, C2, C3, C4 and D2 in the report).

7.2.4 *Line 4: Increase in government debt*

The largest item in Table 7.1 is the WELLBY loss resulting from the increase in government debt, which in the UK totalled around US$36 billion per month. This debt paid for the cost of subsidising businesses no longer allowed to operate, a cost incurred directly because of lockdown policies. That debt will eventually have to be paid back, inevitably crowding out future government investments and services. This materially threatens our future standard of living. If we use the extremely conservative assumption that governments generate one WELLBY for every US$10,000 they spend on such "normal" line items – the actual cost of delivering one WELLBY is probably only half that[225] – then this cost of 'future austerity' works out to **51,400 WELLBYs lost per million citizens per month of lockdown.**

---

[225] On the production costs of a WELLBY, which is what is relevant if we are trying to estimate the effects of future reductions in government services, Frijters and Krekel (2021) write that "the UK Department of Health & Social Care assumes as an internal estimate that it can produce a QALY via the NHS for about £15,000 (Claxton et al 2015; Lomas et al 2019; see also Department of Health, & Department of Education, 2017). We know that an additional year of life in excellent health is worth around six WELLBYs, which, in turn, implies that the NHS currently buys a WELLBY at a rate of £2,500 in 2019 values ... We should mention here that the key studies on the monetary value of a QALY do not really justify that the NHS can buy an additional year of life for £15,000: Claxton et al (2015) looked at improvements in health quality when they estimated that the NHS can buy 1 additional QALY at the price of around £12,936 (in 2008 money) or around £15,000 in 2017 money, using the Consumer Price Index (CPI) as deflator. This is thus their calculated social production costs of 1 QALY via improvements in health, not via life-expectancy. In Appendix 2 of their paper, Claxton et al (2015) also estimate that an additional year of life can be bought by the NHS for about £33,333 in 2009 or about £42,500 in 2017 prices, adjusting for inflation. The authors obtain these estimates by focussing more on mortality-related types of health budgets. There is, therefore, a good argument to be made that the Department of Health and Social Care should differentiate the minimum social production costs for a QALY bought by health improvements from those for a QALY bought by longevity improvements. However, as there is in practice no differentiation, we take £2,500 as our initial threshold for the minimum social production costs of a WELLBY. If we alternatively assume that the NHS produces 2.5 WELLBYs for £15,000 (through health improvements), we obtain a cost per WELLBY of £6,000. In sum, we estimate the minimum social production cost of wellbeing to be between £2,500 and £6,000." (*A Handbook for Wellbeing Policy-Making.* Oxford: Oxford University Press, page xvii.)

7.2.5 Line 5: Pollution

During the early months of COVID lockdowns, one often heard the claim that lockdowns were good for the environment because, surely, CO_2 emissions would be dropping with the reduced economic activity. This turned out not to be true. Many high-energy mass transit systems kept operating, often with hardly any passengers, while private vehicle travel surged as individuals avoided lower-carbon options like public transport and instead drove everywhere in their 'safe' cars.[226] Other pressures on the environment also resulted from lockdowns. For example, lockdowns led to a waste mountain of masks and additional plastic used by shops to wrap purchases separately 'to be safe.' To be conservative, we do not count any net harm from lockdowns in this area.

7.2.6 Line 6: Suicides

The next row of Table 7.1 relates to suicide rates. These were expected by many commentators to rise with unemployment and teenage depression, but this did not turn out to be true in all countries. They may have risen in the US, but not in the UK or many other developed countries. The fair loss to report from the UK lockdowns via suicides is zero.

7.2.7 Line 7: Disruption to education of children

The final element in Table 7.1 quantifies the disruption to the education of children due to school closures that were mandated as part of lockdowns. The significant direct misery that this caused children in the short run is included in the 'satisfaction with life' loss captured

---

[226] A September 2020 article reports that half the respondents in a survey said they are using public transport less often or much less often. Though some people have moved from public transport to clean individual transport such as bicycles, private cars have emerged as the "clear winner" of the shift (Keating, Dave (2020). "Covid Causing Shift From Public Transport To Cars," in *Forbes*, https://archive.ph/Bqp5t). On the other hand, public transport systems continued to be provided despite low levels of use: "the strict lockdown imposed in the UK in March 2020 has led to a 95% decrease in underground journeys in London" (*Source*: Institute of Economic Affairs (2020). "Changes in transport behaviour during the Covid-19 crisis," https://archive.ph/8Eerp).

already, but an additional loss will be incurred in the future as these less-educated people enter the workforce and pay lower taxes. Since government expenditures generate a lot of well-being, this matters. A simple calculation by the Institute for Fiscal Studies in the UK suggested that the lockdowns were costing the value of six months' worth of education, meaning around 100 billion pounds less for governments to spend on things in the future.[227]

That report noted the finding of many studies that the disruption in education is worse at the bottom of the education ladder – that is, among children from lower socio-economic backgrounds. Many of those at the bottom not only failed to advance, but saw their skills deteriorate during lockdowns, as they did little homework and became demotivated.

Taking a conservative estimate that only 20% of the education disrupted by lockdowns was truly lost, the losses in this area work out at **5,714 WELLBYs lost per month of lockdown per one million citizens**. This figure includes only the well-being losses attributable to the reduction in learning quantity during lockdowns, and leaves out the longer-run costs of bad habits and accumulated learning delays that are likely to further depress earnings and hence the government's tax take from the cohort of COVID children in future.

7.3 The result: Lockdown costs overwhelm even the most optimistic estimates of benefits

Even under the unsupportable assumption that lockdowns were able to prevent all COVID deaths, and that such deaths would have been at a level unheard of even in countries like Sweden that did not lock down, lockdowns have imposed a huge net welfare cost in the UK. There are many ways to look at the information provided above.

---

[227] Sibieta, L. (2021). "The crisis in lost learning calls for a massive national policy response," Institute for Fiscal Studies, 1 February 2021, https://www.ifs.org.uk/publications/15291.

- A single month of UK-style lockdown in the developed West is estimated to cost around 250% of the entire loss represented by 0.3% of the population dying of COVID.

- The costs of lockdown were at least 28 times greater during 2020 than any benefits.

- These estimates are based on pessimistic numbers for COVID deaths and highly conservative numbers for the collateral damages. The real collateral damages in the West alone are arguably twice as high. For most nations, lockdowns are now known to have had no clear beneficial effect on the number of COVID cases or deaths. A few exceptions may exist for islands, like New Zealand or Australia, which had significant border closures. However, while COVID deaths might have been delayed in such places, other harms were significant. In most cases, there is no trade-off to be analysed in the area of lockdown policies.[228] There is just loss all around.

The accounting above also does not quantify the costs of lost freedoms, social trust and coherence, or the catastrophic losses suffered in poor countries due to developed nations' lockdowns.

Lockdowns may also have reduced the number of 'normal' pregnancies by 10-20% in some countries,[229] something also not counted in Table 7.1 but that will cause more harm that will be felt for decades.

---

[228] More detailed work is needed that accounts for individual differences among nations in order to confirm that lockdowns do not reduce the spread of a respiratory virus except, potentially, in island nations.

[229] Kearney, Melissa S. and Levine, Phillip (2021). "The coming COVID-19 baby bust is here," Brookings Institute, May 5, 2021, https://bit.ly/39KCzYY. In the UK, "provisional data from the Office for National Statistics suggests there was a temporary decline in babies conceived during the first three months of the first lockdown in 2020, but then the fertility rate rebounded to levels above those seen in previous years." (Berrington, Ann et al (2022). "Effect of lockdowns on birth rates in the UK," in *The Conversation*, 21 April 2022, https://archive.ph/Mkyf6). This pattern of an early reduction and then a rebound in pregnancies probably also occurred during Australian lockdowns. Data on this point from the Australian Bureau of Statistics are presented in a later section for the year to September 2021.

Losses similar to those in Table 7.1 have been found in many Western countries by the authors of dozens of cost-benefit calculations undertaken around the world, in which the damages done by COVID policies to various dimensions of life are translated into a particular single currency, such as WELLBYs, QALYs or dollars, so that like-for-like comparisons can be made across categories.

8. Benefits of Australia's lockdowns

In constructing my cost-benefit analysis of Australia's lockdown policies, I give the government significant benefit of the doubt. I use conservative assumptions – assumptions biased in favour of finding that lockdowns were a good idea – to estimate the benefits of lockdowns and related policies that were implemented in Australian regions in stops and starts from late March 2020 to the end of 2021. Likewise, I actively seek to use the lowest reasonable cost estimates.

A schematic outline of the potential benefits from Australia's lockdowns, including their stated goal of reducing COVID-related suffering and deaths, but also allowing for other potential benefits, is provided in Figure 8.1.

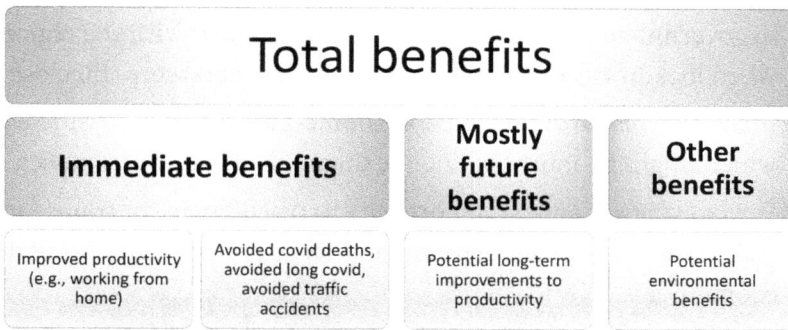

Figure 8.1: Schematic depiction of potential benefits from Australia's lockdowns

8.1 Benefit 1: Economic benefits of lockdowns

While they decimated some businesses, such as many operating in sectors like tourism and the arts, lockdowns have been great for other types of businesses. They have changed the professional norms around working from home, potentially saving individual workers commuting time and other costs, and have forced experimentation that has resulted in the discovery of more efficient ways of conducting knowledge work (e.g., videocalls for committee meetings that used to be held in-person).

The kinds of economic benefits that have likely emerged due to lockdowns include:

- Shifts to working from home across most ICT-enabled businesses, and re-designing of business models across the board to minimise physical human interaction – leading potentially to short-run increases in productivity. However, some of the benefits to productivity from the changes to the way knowledge work is conducted may be short-lived, with reports that working from home causes stress[230] and potentially reduced creativity.[231]

- Positive spillovers of re-designed business models to the re-design of cities, though likely not much, since agglomeration effects and physical interaction are likely to remain important for productivity in the longer run.

- Some of the loss in domestic tourism revenue was recouped due to government programs and a rush for people to visit the regions when lockdowns lifted but international borders were still closed.

- Increased resources devoted to home-based online businesses, which might be more productive than out-of-home businesses.

- Fewer expenses and an opportunity to pay off debt for some Australian families, meaning more capacity to spend in support of the economy.

- The earlier retirement of some older workers may have provided opportunities for the younger and potentially more productive generation.

As a rule, these benefits accrued more to individuals in more well-paid, white-collar occupations, leading to greater economic inequality as people in less-well paid occupations, such as those requiring manual work, suffered more.

---

[230] E.g., *The Guardian* (2021). "Revealed: rise in stress among those working from home," 4 July 2021, https://bit.ly/3MCUWh6.

[231] E.g., McGraw Hill Education (2021). "Microsoft Study Says Working from Home Decreases Teamwork and Creativity," https://bit.ly/3NCAbSG.

Some of these benefits or comparable levels of benefits from other developments might have accrued even without lockdowns, as people chose voluntarily to shift to new ways of working or discovered other innovations.

The most straightforward way to assess the importance of these benefits in the short run is to look at the change in real GDP per capita during lockdowns. GDP per capita fell in three quarters since the start of 2020 (Figure 8.2), and any positive effect on productivity in the short run is already reflected in those figures. In other words, without whatever productivity increases were brought by lockdowns, the reduction in GDP per capita observed in these three quarters would have been even greater.

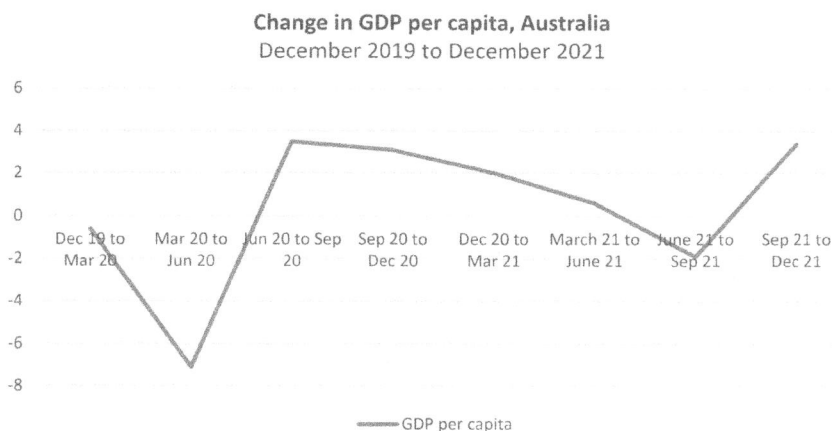

Change in GDP per capita, Australia
December 2019 to December 2021

Figure 8.2: Three-quarters of negative GDP per capita growth were observed during 2020 and 2021[232]

Another way to look at the impact of lockdowns on current economic health is to consider overall household final consumption expenditure in the recent past (as shown in Figure 8.3), as a proxy for household buying capacity, and compare this against historical trends. Two potential trendlines are shown in Figure 8.3 that could be used to extrapolate consumer expenditure post-COVID. Regardless of which is used, even by December 2021 household expenditure

---

[232] This chart has been constructed from relevant ABS data releases, with older releases considered more accurate.

had not caught up with a simple projection of pre-COVID historical trends. This indicates that any short-run gains in the areas above due to lockdowns were outweighed by losses.

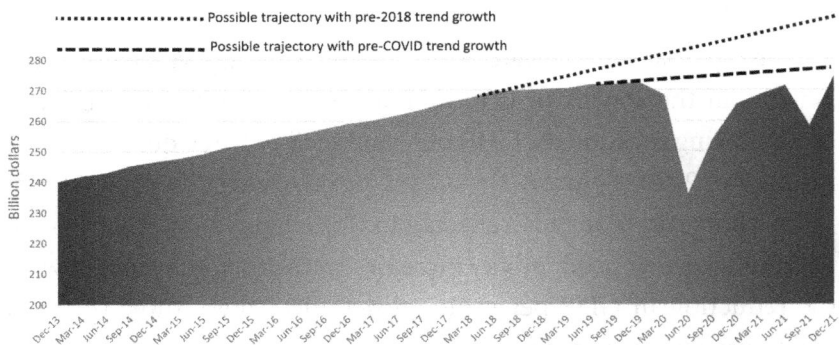

Figure 8.3: Household final consumption expenditure, volume measures, seasonally adjusted, 2013-2021[233]

In terms of the potential for longer-run economic benefits arising from lockdowns, there are reasons to expect negative benefits in some areas (e.g., reduced levels of international students and tourism, reduced motivation for work and/or labour force participation) as well as some continuing positive benefits (e.g., online committee meetings), relative to the counterfactual of what Australia would have had if it had followed the pre-2020 policy playbook in managing COVID. How these effects will balance out in future years is unknown and probably never will be known, given the complexity of estimating the unseen long-run counterfactual scenario. As a result, in this report I assume zero net long-run economic benefits of lockdowns.

8.2 Benefit 2: Improved well-being from lockdowns for those in Australia

The mental health of some people may well have improved from lockdowns. Some fortunate people were able to increase the amount of quality time spent with their family during lockdowns while working from home, and the net income of some households increased, leading to upward pressure on life satisfaction. Some students may have

---

[233] Australian Bureau of Statistics (2022). Australian National Accounts: National Income, Expenditure and Product, 2 March 2022, https://bit.ly/3wFCEFq.

also enjoyed home schooling, even though for others it was stress-ful. Any well-being benefits accruing to a fraction of the population experiencing lockdowns are included in the average life satisfaction changes estimated from surveys taken during lockdown periods, which I discuss later in a chapter on costs. In other words, without these benefits for some people, the short-run loss in total well-being brought about by lockdowns would have been even higher.

8.3 Benefit 3: Improved health and longevity outcomes (including increases in population)

Did births increase or decrease during lockdowns, and how many potential deaths from COVID were averted?

8.3.1 *Effect on births*

Lockdowns are not designed as a policy to increase births – that is not even their secondary or tertiary policy objective – but they could potentially have indirect effects that increase births.

(i) Direct effects that decrease births

Some Australian couples will have been separated due to sudden border closures, and the efforts of some young people to meet a part-ner and start a family will have been stymied by disruptions to typi-cal dating activities, both of which will have put downward pressure on births. Marriages plummeted from 113,815 in 2019 to 78,989 in 2020.[234] Whether births that might have occurred earlier under nor-mal circumstances will now occur later in the lives of these couples remains to be seen.

Stress and lack of adequate access to maternity care may have caused more miscarriages and stillbirths than usual. On 3 November 2020, it was reported that in the UK, "Stillbirths doubled during first wave of Covid-19 pandemic amid fears that mothers were delayed

---

[234] Australian Bureau of Statistics (2021). Marriages and Divorces, Australia, 24 Novem-ber 2021, https://bit.ly/3wB0d20.

from seeking NHS care."[235] There are similar reports for Australia.[236] Although the number of stillbirths is not large (40 stillbirths were reported between April and June compared to 24 in the same period in 2019), miscarriages are more common.

(ii) Direct effects that increase births

Unintended but direct policy effects of lockdowns on increased births could have occurred through reduced access to contraception methods mediated by the medical system. We do not have precise information on these effects, and I therefore ignore them.

IVF treatments have experienced a strong positive trend in recent years. 14,355 babies were born in 2018 through IVF treatment performed in Australia,[237] and this figure grew in 2019: "88,929 IVF cycles started in 2019 (81,049 in Australia and 7880 in New Zealand), leading to 16,310 babies born through the treatment."[238]

IVF was deemed "non-essential" during the first month of lockdowns,[239] meaning that fewer IVF babies will have been conceived during that period. While we do not have a precise estimate of this effect, IVF cycles might have seen a net increase during the full span of 2020 and 2021. Illustratively, a total of 6071 WA women underwent IVF in 2020-21, an increase of 1230 on the previous year.[240] If the WA experience is replicated nationally, an additional 3,000 babies could have been born in Australia through the IVF route, or say, 5,000 during the two-year period 2020 and 2021. Any such increase would show up in overall births data.

---

[235] *Daily Mail*, UK (2 November 2020). "Stillbirths DOUBLED during first wave of Covid-19 pandemic amid fears that mothers were delayed from seeking NHS care," https://bit.ly/3wP8Nui.

[236] *ABC News* (25 November 2021). "Stillbirth rates rose in Melbourne's COVID-19 lockdown, despite dropping overall in past three years," https://bit.ly/3PCoz3V.

[237] University of New South Wales (2 September 2020). "Almost one in 20 babies in Australia born through IVF," https://bit.ly/3Nr1CPq.

[238] *NewsGP* (22 September 2021). "IVF success rate increasing in Australia," https://bit.ly/3PEzoCA.

[239] A temporary ban was imposed from mid-March 2020 to 28 April 2020 (City Fertility. "IVF treatment to recommence across Australia," https://bit.ly/3MIC4gW).

[240] Elton, Charlotte (2021). "IVF boom attributed to effects of pandemic," in *The West Australian*, 15 October 2021, https://bit.ly/3lAxRjk.

(iii) Indirect effects

An increase in economic uncertainty may have a variety of effects on fertility. In the short term, people may have fewer children as they fear being unable to afford the children's education and care. With heightened stress, prospective parents may also become less fecund. If poverty is expected to be chronic, birth rates might increase, as seen in developing nations. Lockdowns might also have increased births through increasing the time spent by workers with their intimate partners and strengthening people's focus on their families. Overall, there is no obvious theoretical basis on which to expect a significant net indirect effect either way of lockdowns on fertility.

Any net impact of lockdowns on fertility would show up only from the December 2020 quarter, and relevant ABS data have recently started to emerge.

1) ABS data as at September 2021 (released on 17 March 2022)[241] suggest that conceptions decreased during the first month or two of lockdowns, then normalised, and then began to rise. A review of recorded births in Australia since March 2020[242] shows that in the year to September 2021, births per quarter increased by 7,700, or 2.6%. Longer-term data series on quarterly births in Australia display significant volatility, so caution is needed in interpreting any short-term variation.

2) In the year ending 30 September 2021, Australia welcomed 303,700 births. This does not stand out when compared against pre-COVID data. In the year 2020 for example, 294,369 births were recorded, most of which were of babies conceived prior to March 2020.[243] The total fertility rate (TFR) in 2019-20 was 1.609,[244] in line

---

[241] *Source*: Australian Bureau of Statistics (2022). National, state and territory population, 17 March 2022, https://bit.ly/3wLYjeU.

[242] *Source*: Table 10 of datacube 31010do001_202109 National, state and territory population, Sep 2021 from ABS: https://archive.ph/5jlo2.

[243] Australian Bureau of Statistics (2021). "Australian fertility rate hits record low," 8 December 2021, https://bit.ly/3yUylbU.

[244] *Source*: Table 10 of datacube 31010do001_202109 National, state and territory population, Sep 2021 from https://archive.ph/5jlo2.

with the trend since 2008-2009.[245] In 2020-21, the TFR increased marginally to 1.618, still consistent with the trend.

3) A longer-term perspective on births in Australia is provided in Figure 8.4.

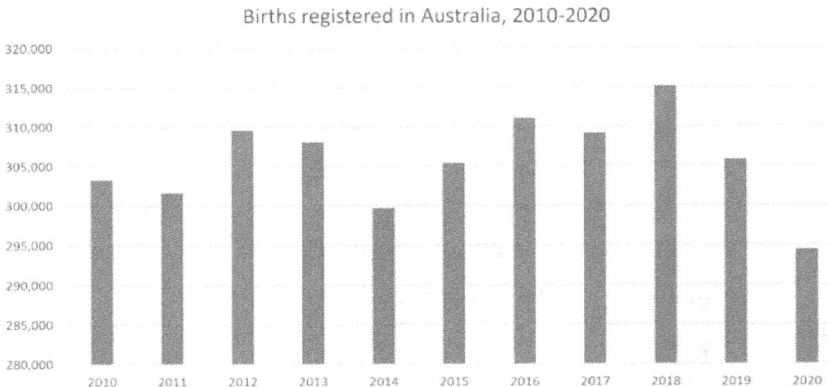

Births registered in Australia, 2010-2020

Figure 8.4: The number of births in Australia, 2010-2020[246]

The distribution of births is dependent on many factors beyond the TFR. While the TFR has declined monotonically in Australia from 2015 to 2020, Figure 8.4 shows that the number of births varies substantially across years. Births are also driven by factors such as the population structure, including the size of the cohort which is passing through its reproductive stage.

When this longer-term perspective (with extreme variation in births) is superimposed on the short-term data for the pandemic period, Australia's 303,700 births in the year to September 2021 do not stand out as exceptional. Births have exhibited similar rebounds from dips in the past (e.g., between 2014 and 2015, and between 2017 and 2018), despite the TFR declining almost monotonically throughout.

Since the total number of births in Australia is relatively small and subject to significant natural variation, which would apply equally to

---

[245] McDonald, Peter (2021). "Australian fertility trends: a sociodemographic perspective," O&G Magazine, Vol. 23 No.1, Autumn 2021, https://archive.ph/0oaAz.

[246] *Source*: Spreadsheet – Births registered, 1932 to 2020(a), from ABS: https://bit.ly/3ySppni. Data for 2021 will become available from the ABS in December 2022.

the counterfactual no-lockdown scenario, I am unable confidently to attribute the observed increase in births during 2020-21 to lockdowns for the purpose of this report. I therefore incorporate a net zero estimated effect of lockdowns on births.

If more conclusive data emerge, it may become appropriate to update the lockdown effects counted in this CBA with some proportion of the observed changes in births. One approach would be to confirm whether the effect seen in Australia is also evident in other locked down nations but not in places with fewer restrictions, like Sweden.

Even if an increase in births were to be attributed to lockdowns in the future, it would not make lockdowns suitable as a policy intended to increase Australia's population. As discussed below, the net impact of lockdowns on the Australian population count is negative and hence counts as a cost rather than a benefit, because of a dramatic decline in immigration.

8.3.2 COVID deaths postponed by lockdowns

Although evidence is emerging that lockdowns globally did not reduce COVID deaths, or did so very marginally, I assume that some lives, mostly of the elderly, were potentially extended by Australia's strict lockdowns – particularly since it is an island nation that opted to close borders. At the same time, many life-years of the elderly that could have been enjoyed if there had been a policy focus on aged care facilities and other vulnerable groups were probably lost due to the ill-targeted efforts of government.[247]

I consider below two methods to estimate COVID deaths postponed by Australia's lockdowns.

- First, I use Sweden, a country that implemented no lockdowns or total border closures, as a comparator. What happened in Sweden is an imperfect but plausible proxy for what happens in an ideal

---

[247] As previously discussed, lockdowns represent an abandonment of the standard risk-based approach to public policy. They apply interventions to people regardless of their actual risk of harm, instead of focusing interventions on high-risk cohorts.

COVID world without lockdowns, but with targeted policies consistent with pre-2020 pandemic management plans.

• Second, I extrapolate based on reported COVID deaths from selected countries other than Sweden that also had relatively low levels of restrictions.

Using a combination of these two estimation methods, I find that the upper limit of COVID deaths postponed by Australia's lockdowns is **9,951** for the two years of 2020 and 2021 combined, as detailed below.

8.3.2.1 *Extrapolating from Sweden's excess COVID death count*

There would be no public health emergency if COVID only caused deaths equivalent to what typical respiratory viruses cause in an average year. In an average year, for example, the endemic flu virus causes up to 650,000 deaths globally.[248]

What matters is excess deaths caused by COVID beyond what is "normal" (i.e., including respiratory viruses like the flu) since that is the best measure of the magnitude of the pandemic. Reported COVID death statistics do not compare the harms that COVID is causing to what would be expected without COVID, nor to the total annual deaths in the nation. This lack of contextualisation implicitly exaggerates the magnitude of the pandemic.

We can split reported COVID deaths into three: (a) Category A, being reported deaths *with* COVID but from other than respiratory causes, (b) Category B, being reported deaths *from* COVID over and above the expected (normal) respiratory virus deaths, and (c) Category C, being reported respiratory deaths from COVID which displaced other "normal" respiratory (e.g., flu) deaths in the average year.

Category A is the most pernicious, as it most directly exaggerates the perception of threat from COVID among the public, but to isolate and exclude the reported "COVID" deaths in this category one

---

[248] World Health Organization. Global Influenza Programme, https://bit.ly/3NsnERU.

would need detailed information about each death. However, a way to derive a meaningful calculation for Category B will be illustrated using Sweden's data.

Sweden is of interest since it did roughly what Australia was supposed to have done as prescribed in its official pandemic plans when facing a virus like COVID. It implemented minimally appropriate restrictions, almost all of them voluntary. Had Australia not imposed lockdowns, one might argue that it would have had population-adjusted deaths similar in number to what Sweden experienced.

For several reasons, this is a pessimistic counterfactual. Australia's population is younger than Sweden's;[249] Australia's population has higher exposure to sunlight, so probably less vitamin D deficiency, than Sweden's; and Australia's aged care homes are not as dense as those in Sweden (discussed further below). For reasons like this, plus the "dry tinder" effect from the mild 2019 Swedish flu season, the death rate in Sweden from COVID likely over-estimates the death rate Australia would have seen under the no-lockdown counterfactual.

I assume here that all excess deaths in Sweden in 2020 and 2021 were caused by COVID, even though there must have been at least some excess deaths for other reasons (for example, due to reductions in visits to GPs and hospitals by people too scared to venture there).

Despite criticisms that its elderly were inadequately cocooned at the start of the pandemic, Sweden ended up with relatively few excess deaths in 2020. For instance, Figure 8.5 shows that if the dry tinder effect of 2019[250] is combined with the presence of COVID in 2020 and 2021, the mortality rate drops close to trend: 90.6 per 10,000 is the average mortality rate across 2020 and 2021, which is the same as the 2018 mortality rate. Its 2020 death rate – even if taken in isolation

---

[249] https://data.worldbank.org/indicator/SP.POP.65UP.TO.ZS), World Bank, "Population ages 65 and above (% of total population)."

[250] "Sweden's chief epidemiologist has partly blamed the country's high coronavirus death toll on mild flu outbreaks in recent winters" (*CNBC*. "Sweden's high coronavirus death toll could be linked to mild flu seasons, chief scientist says," 23 September 2020, https://bit.ly/3aaEc2p).

– was lower than the average death rate from 2000-2021. Such "business as usual" results were achieved without any lockdowns, mandatory masks, quarantines, or extended border closures. This suggests very few, if any, deaths in Category B.

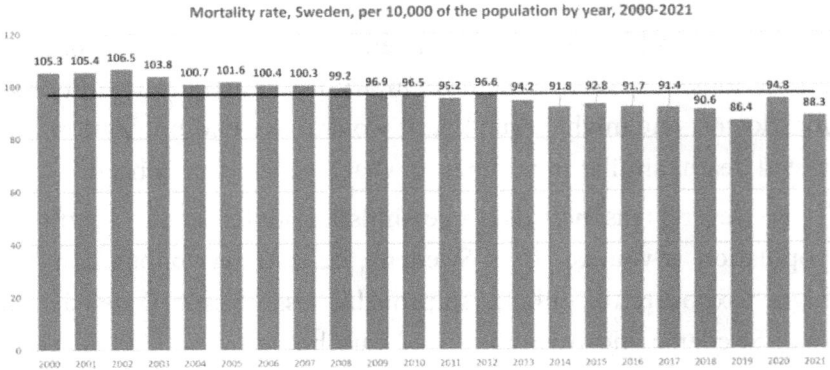

Mortality rate, Sweden, per 10,000 of the population by year, 2000-2021

Figure 8.5: The death rate of Sweden over the past 20 years: COVID was evidently not a severe pandemic[251]

Some people have pointed out that Sweden's reported COVID death rate has been higher than that of its neighbours. Worldometer data on COVID deaths per million as at 4 July 2022 show the following: Sweden 1867, Finland 877, and Norway 606. However, any attempts to use this as an alleged "smoking gun" of Sweden's "failure" to justify lockdowns are fraught, for several reasons.

a) While the Oxford Stringency Index ("OxCGRT" hereafter) is an imperfect measure of the severity of COVID-excused restrictions implemented by governments, it shows that neighbouring Scandinavian nations had COVID policies that were broadly similar to Sweden's. Jon Miltimore notes that "Sweden's government response stringency never reached 50, peaking at about 46 from late April to early June [2020]." At the same time, "Norway's lockdown stringency has been less than 40 since early June [2020], and fell all the way to 28.7 in September and October. Finland's lockdown stringency followed a similar pattern, floating around the mid to low 30s for most

251 Statistics Sweden (SCB). "Mortality rate per 1,000 of the mean population by age and sex. Year 2000–2020," https://bit.ly/3MEgmdX.

of the second half of the year, before creeping back up to 41 around Halloween."[252] All three countries, therefore, had comparatively low levels of restrictions.

b) Several factors pushed COVID deaths higher in Sweden than in its neighbours. These include the "dry tinder" effect of a mild flu season in Sweden in 2019 already mentioned, and a more vulnerable elderly population than in neighbouring countries due to features of its aged care sector. As reported by Swedish economist Fredrik Erixon: "Sweden's nursing homes have for a long time been dangerous places for their residents during the flu season…The country has about 12,150 nursing home beds per million citizens compared to 7,800 in Norway. Each nursing home also has more residents. A virus that is spread in a Swedish nursing home will kill more people than in a Norwegian home."[253]

One reason why Sweden's death count was not larger during the COVID era is that panic kills. Harsh policies like workplace closures, lockdowns (including internal restrictions on movement) and forced masking cause a sense of panic. Negative spillovers on health then ensue, from reduced immunity due to stress and avoidance of sunlight to an increase in obesity and diabetes, thus making the population more vulnerable to COVID fatalities than it would have been otherwise. Sweden's government messaging was calming and retained a broad focus on mental health and public health, while most other nations' messaging, including Australia's, often frightened their populations and drove people into anxiety and despair.

Using deaths in 2017-2019 in Sweden as a baseline, Nobel laureate Michael Levitt has found that 2,996 excess deaths occurred in Sweden in 2020,[254] representing around 3% of its expected annual deaths.

[252] Foundation for Economic Freedom (13 November 2020). "How Finland and Norway Proved Sweden's Approach to COVID-19 Works," https://bit.ly/3wCH5BU.

[253] Erixon, Fredrik (2020). "The crisis in Sweden's care homes," in *The Spectator*, 21 April 2020, https://bit.ly/39Q41F2.

[254] Tweet dated 25 February 2021 by Michael Levitt, https://bit.ly/38BA0sk.

I consider Levitt's analysis to be a credible approximation. While Figure 8.5 suggests it would be reasonable to attribute no excess deaths in Sweden to COVID, for this study I will be conservative and take Michael Levitt's estimate as the upper bound for the potential size of Category B in Sweden.

Extrapolating Michael Levitt's estimate of 2,996 excess deaths in Sweden to Australia's population yields a possible **7,436** excess deaths during 2020 for Australia in a COVID world (2,996 x (25.69/10.35)), were we not to have imposed lockdowns. Again, because of differences between Sweden and Australia in factors such as age structure, latitude, and features of the aged care sectors, this number should be considered an upper bound.

In 2021, Sweden *prima facie* had no excess deaths, with overall mortality at 88.3 per 10,000, the lowest in the country's recorded history. However, in that year, Sweden also reported 5,344 COVID deaths.[255] This suggests that its reported COVID deaths in 2021 merely displaced normal respiratory virus deaths (i.e., they fell into Category C). This means that effectively none, or very few, additional deaths were caused by COVID in Sweden in 2021 that would not otherwise have happened. Regardless, to be conservative, I assume that COVID caused an extra 1000 deaths in Sweden in 2021. Proportionately, Australia would then have had around **2,468** (1,000 x (25.75/10.43)) excess COVID deaths in 2021 in a no-lockdown policy regime.

Over the course of two years (2020 and 2021), therefore, a conservative estimate is that Australia would have had **9,904** excess respiratory virus deaths because of COVID in the absence of lockdowns.

8.3.2.2 *Extrapolating from the COVID death count of nations with less stringent policies*

Countries apart from Sweden also took a broadly risk-based approach, similar to what Swedish public health leader Anders Tegnell articulated and implemented, and did not create mass-scale panic.

---

[255] https://www.worldometers.info/coronavirus/country/sweden/.

In this section I identify such countries using the OxCGRT database and then use their COVID death counts to construct a second counterfactual comparator for Australia using which the potential benefits brought by lockdowns can be estimated.[256]

The Stringency Index created by the OxCGRT project of the Blavatnik School of Government at the University of Oxford is not tethered to risk-based public health practices and outcomes. It tracks the various restrictions that governments enacted without distinguishing between countries that followed zero-covid policies from those that took a risk-based mitigation stance. The design of the Stringency Index averages arithmetically 9 ordinally created variables that are in many cases coded in a manner which does not capture the likely impact of a policy on people's well-being. For example, it fails to distinguish between the collateral impacts of recommendations and those of police-enforced mandates.

Nonetheless, I use the OxCGRT database in this report by combining the four variables labelled C2, C7, C6 and H6 (Workplace Closures, Restrictions on Internal Movement, Stay-at-Home Requirements and Facial Coverings)[257] to capture the policy stance of a nation. By sorting countries on the sum of these four variables, where higher values indicate fewer restrictions, I identify 6 nations of a million or more people from the developed world (Figure 8.6) which had relatively less onerous policies. In this list Sweden is close to the top, indicating the reasonableness of this ranking. I then use reported outcomes in these six nations to estimate the deaths that could have occurred in Australia without lockdowns.[258]

---

[256] Blavatnik School of Government, University of Oxford, "COVID-19 Government Response Tracker," https://bit.ly/3G9o9xE.

[257] OxCGRT. Codebook for the Oxford Covid-19 Government Response Tracker (Codebook version 3.7, 11 March 2022), https://bit.ly/3LCnF4y.

[258] I have excluded Iceland and Greenland because their populations are very small (Iceland has 366,425 people, Greenland 56,367). While future work may select different sets of comparator nations to construct this alternative counterfactual, I can see no selection that would cause the overall conclusion reached in this report, i.e., that lockdowns were not worth their costs, to change.

Figure 8.6: The OxCGRT database sorted on the sum of C2, C6, C7 and H6

Country	C2	C6	C7	H6	Sum
Grenada	0	0	0	261	261
Nicaragua	0	0	0	528	528
Tanzania	21	21	21	896	959
Vanuatu	460	207	269	257	1193
Burundi	400	28	119	798	1345
Kiribati	257	428	188	512	1385
Faeroe Islands	1007	189	69	484	1749
Macao	300	0	33	1578	1911
Belarus	163	503	0	1292	1958
Sweden	723	581	333	330	1967
Iceland	842	0	0	1177	2019
Greenland	448	305	256	1088	2097
Finland	1052	406	92	765	2315
Niger	169	10	103	2108	2390
Estonia	996	165	268	1227	2656
Cameroon	207	0	309	2208	2724
Sudan	818	394	334	1239	2785
Taiwan	532	138	204	1926	2800
Gambia	485	338	180	1827	2830
Norway	1113	383	427	980	2903

Table 8.1 displays data assembled for these six nations from Worldometer and supplementary internet searches.

Country	COVID deaths as at 31 December 2020	COVID deaths as at 31 December 2021	COVID deaths in 2021	Population in 2020 (million)	Population in 2021 (million)	Death/m 2020	Deaths/m 2021
Belarus	1,424	5,578	4,154	9.399	9.43	151.5	440.5
Sweden	9,904	15,347	5,443	10.35	10.43	956.9	521.9
Finland	561	1,564	1,003	5.531	5.5	101.4	182.4
Estonia	229	1,932	1,703	1.331	1.32	172.1	1290.2
Taiwan	7	850	843	23.57	23.6	0.3	35.7
Norway	440	1,334	894	5.379	5.39	81.8	165.9
Total	12,565	26,605	14,040	56	56	226.2	252.2

Table 8.1: COVID deaths in nations with broadly risk-based policies

Overall, low-restriction nations reported fewer COVID deaths than other nations. However, these counts have not been adjusted using information on excess deaths, as done for the case of Sweden above, and no local factors are adjusted for. Taiwan's record is an outlier and suggests another line of future analysis: determining the costs and benefits for island nations of international border closures *per se* in combatting disease.

The data in Table 8.1 yields an average of 226.2 COVID deaths per million in 2020 and 252.2 COVID deaths per million in 2021 across these six countries. Extrapolating to Australia, this would equate to 226.2 x 25.69 = **5,810** maximum COVID deaths in Australia in 2020 and 252.2 x 25.75 = **6,494** maximum COVID deaths in Australia in 2021. This yields a maximum total of **12,304** COVID deaths that Australia might have had without lockdowns in 2020 and 2021.

8.3.3 *Long COVID avoided by lockdowns*

Since the publication of *The Great Covid Panic*, more evidence has accumulated about the prevalence and impact of long COVID.

On 24 September 2021 the following was reported in *The Times*:

> Professor Sir John Bell, regius professor of medicine at Oxford University, said that long Covid was "more complicated than people assume" and that "the incidence is much, much lower than people had anticipated". His comments follow data from the Office for National Statistics (ONS) which suggests that half of people suffering from long Covid may not have it.[259]

An 8 November 2021 study delivered controversial findings suggesting a lack of stronger long-COVID-like symptoms in antibody-positive French people relative to antibody-negative French people:[260]

---

[259] Gibbons, Katie (2021). "Long Covid is overblown and often something else, says Oxford professor," in *The Times*, 24 September 2021, https://bit.ly/3MGBhwW.

[260] Matta, Joane et al (2021). "Association of Self-reported COVID-19 Infection and SARS-CoV-2 Serology Test Results With Persistent Physical Symptoms Among French Adults During the COVID-19 Pandemic," in *JAMA Intern Med*, Doi:10.1001/jamainternmed.2021.6454 published online 8 November 2021, https://jamanetwork.com/journals/jamainternalmedicine/fullarticle/2785832.

Researchers found that people who believed they had had COVID, whether or not they had had a positive test, were more likely to report long-term symptoms.[261]

This is consistent with the findings of a 23 September 2020 report in JAMA which found that "[m]any long haulers never had laboratory confirmation of COVID-19."[262]

It appears likely that a proportion of self-reported long COVID sufferers are suffering for reasons unrelated to a COVID infection.

According to a 3 March 2022 report by the ONS, UK, "[a]n estimated 1.5 million people living in private households in the UK (2.4% of the population) were experiencing self-reported long COVID (symptoms persisting for more than four weeks after the first suspected coronavirus (COVID-19) infection that were not explained by something else) as of 31 January 2022."[263] It is also now believed that vaccination will not prevent long COVID.[264]

A key question for this report is how to estimate the welfare loss from long COVID averted by lockdowns. My co-authors and I used an estimate of long COVID losses equivalent to 5% of the losses represented by COVID deaths in *The Great Covid Panic*. For Australia in the present report, I use an updated figure of **2%**. This update is in part because we have now had more time to observe the recovery patterns of long COVID cases. The most updated evidence indicates that most of those who do get long COVID are not significantly handicapped in their normal productive activities, and that most

---

[261] *Medical Express* (12 November 2021). "Mind over matter? Long Covid study sparks controversy," https://archive.ph/KUnZO.

[262] https://jamanetwork.com/journals/jama/fullarticle/2771111, Rubin, Rita (2020). "As Their Numbers Grow, COVID-19 'Long Haulers' Stump Experts," *JAMA*, 2020;324(14):1381-1383. Doi:10.1001/jama.2020.17709.

[263] Office for National Statistics. "Prevalence of ongoing symptoms following coronavirus (COVID-19) infection in the UK: 3 March 2022," https://bit.ly/3MD13lr.

[264] At Swiss Policy Research ("Covid Vaccine Adverse Events," https://archive.ph/4O5q0) it is claimed that "In general, vaccination cannot prevent "long covid," as vaccination cannot prevent infection and mild covid (which is sufficient to trigger long covid). According to a US study, vaccination reduced the risk of developing long covid symptoms by only 13%. Furthermore, covid vaccination may itself cause long covid symptoms, likely due to an immune reaction to the coronavirus spike protein."

cases that would measurably impact life satisfaction resolve within three months and the great majority of the remainder within a year.[265] With some accommodation, many employers and employees are largely able to manage the disability caused by long COVID.[266]

8.3.4 *Other deaths avoided by lockdowns*

Lockdowns might have avoided some additional deaths for reasons wholly unrelated to respiratory disease. Plausibly, with fewer people going about their usual daily activities, fewer young people may have been killed by gang and other violence, and fewer traffic deaths may have occurred. There is some evidence that this might have occurred, such as:

- An analysis of crime reports from 27 cities in Europe, Asia and the Americas found overall urban crime fell by more than a third while lockdowns were in place and then steadily climbed back up when restrictions were lifted.[267]
- Traffic volume dropped sharply during the COVID-19 pandemic, which was associated with a significant drop in traffic accidents globally and a reduction in road deaths in 32 out of 36 countries in April 2020 as compared with April 2019.[268]

Figure 8.7 shows road fatalities in Australia for the past two years. Given the downward trend since 2016, it is hard to deduce any significant reduction in traffic deaths attributable to lockdowns *per se*. The absolute numbers of road collision deaths potentially avoided are miniscule in the grand scheme – at most 9 deaths avoided on net

[265] Hensher, Martin et al (2021). "We calculated the impact of 'long COVID' as Australia opens up. Even without Omicron, we're worried," Deakin University, 16 December 2021, https://bit.ly/39JeQs5; Swiss Policy Research. Post-Acute Covid and Long Covid, https://bit.ly/3MD1egB.

[266] *Time*. "Back-to-Office Pressure Is Creating a Crisis for Long COVID Patients," 28 March 2022, https://bit.ly/3wBfjpf.

[267] *The Guardian* (2021). "Urban crime plummets during lockdowns in cities around world," 2 June 2021, https://bit.ly/3yUD0L6.

[268] Yasin, Yasin J. et al (2021). "Global impact of COVID-19 pandemic on road traffic collisions," in *World Journal of Emergency Surgery*, 16, Article number: 51, 28 September 2021. https://bit.ly/3GbtswL.

per month in 2020 if we naively attribute the entire 2019-2020 reduction shown in Figure 8.7 to lockdowns imposed in 2020. Making this conservative choice yields 77 lives saved, and a similar calculation for 2021 (against 2019) yields 22 lives saved.

12 month total

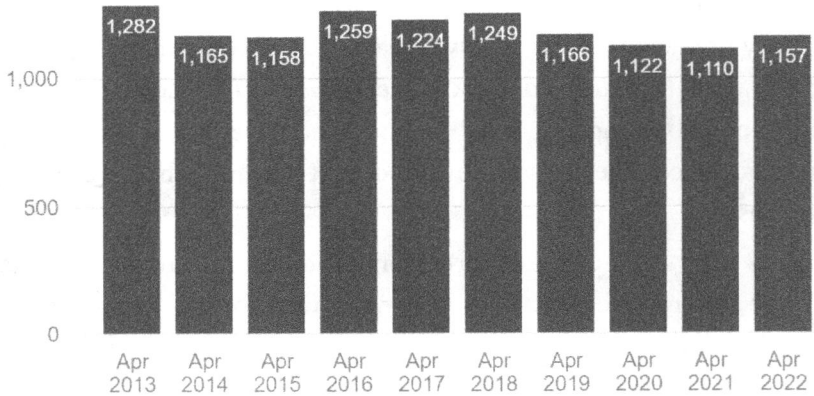

Figure 8.7: Road fatalities in Australia[269]

On crime, the ABS reported that "In 2020, there were 396 victims of homicide and related offences recorded by the police. This was a decrease of 19 victims from 2019."[270] A longer-term chart of the homicide rate per 100,000 population, 1990-2018 from Macrotrends[271] shows a declining trend for the past 30 years, so once again it is hard to tease out the specific contribution of lockdowns to the decline seen in 2020. Nevertheless, I naively attribute all of these 19 lives saved to lockdowns in 2020 and assume the same would have held in 2021.

Therefore, I conservatively assume a savings of 96 (77+19) lives in 2020 and 41 (22+19) lives in 2021 by lockdowns that would otherwise have occurred due to traffic accidents and homicides.

---

[269] *Source*: https://archive.ph/17Pql, Bureau of Infrastructure and Transport Research Economics.

[270] Australian Bureau of Statistics (2022). Recorded Crime – Victims, 24 June 2021, https://bit.ly/3wMvrU5.

[271] Macrotrends. "Australia Murder/Homicide Rate 1990-2022," https://bit.ly/3MFlWwB.

8.3.5 *Estimate of deaths avoided in Australia*

Now we can assemble an estimate of the maximum COVID deaths avoided by lockdowns in Australia.

a) Considering the results from the two methods above of constructing the counterfactual number of COVID deaths (a comparison with Sweden's deaths, versus a comparison with deaths reported in a group of nations with relatively few lockdowns and mandates), I continue my conservative approach by taking the higher figure of **12,304 COVID deaths avoided.** This is a high-end estimate of the number of deaths that might have been caused by COVID in Australia during 2020 and 2021 but were not, due to lockdowns and related policies.

Yet, not all these COVID deaths were in fact avoided. There were 947 COVID deaths in Australia in 2020,[272] and Worldometer reports that Australia cumulatively had 2,353 COVID deaths as at 31 December 2021, which means it had 1,406 COVID deaths in 2021. This means that at most a further **9,951** COVID deaths (12304 – 2353) might have been avoided by the Australian lockdowns.[273] Worldometer data indicate that Australia has had 10,040 COVID deaths during 2022 as at 4 July 2022. This suggests that a large fraction, if not all, of the roughly 10,000 people whose lives were potentially "saved" from a COVID death in Australia by lockdowns in 2020 and 2021 succumbed a year or two later to COVID anyway.

b) To this I add the value of **131** (96+41) deaths prevented by lockdowns due to reductions in homicides and traffic fatalities. Such deaths should be weighted differently than COVID deaths in the overall well-being benefit calculation, since victims of homicides and traffic accidents generally are much younger than COVID victims. I assume conservatively that the average death through these means is of a person with 50 years of healthy life left to live.

---

[272] https://www.worldometers.info/coronavirus/country/australia/.

[273] My round-figure estimate in the early version of this report, submitted to the Public Accounts and Estimates Committee (PAEC) of the Victorian Parliament on 12 August 2020 and excluding any homicide or traffic fatality reductions, was that 10,000 COVID deaths may have potentially been avoided by lockdowns (https://bit.ly/3wEGAHK).

Summing up yields 11,392 deaths (9,951 COVID deaths and 131 non-COVID deaths) potentially avoided by lockdowns during 2020 and 2021.

8.4 Benefit 4: Other benefits from lockdowns

A lower impact on the environment via reduced pollution by not traveling as much is often cited as a potential environmental benefit of lockdowns. As my co-authors and I showed in *The Great Covid Panic*, any reduction in pollution by road travel was at least partly offset by:

- continued operation of mass transit (buses, trains); and
- increased use of private vehicles (which led to a huge demand for second-hand vehicles) as people avoided less polluting mass transit and opted to drive in their 'safe' cars.[274]

There are two main types of atmospheric pollutants: particulate matter and toxic gases, and CO_2. Data indicates that the trend of a decline in CO_2 emissions in Australia since around 2009 was further strengthened in 2020.[275]

Contributing to this was a decline in air travel. Australia had even fewer flights than the global average for most of 2020 (National Greenhouse Inventory, December 2020 update[276]).

Lockdowns may have resulted in improved situations for wildlife, since many national parks were closed to the public during this period, or people were not able to access these habitats, allowing wildlife to be at lower risk from human disturbance. However, reduced stewardship by humans of natural habitats because those humans were locked down may have mitigated this benefit.

---

[274] After a few months of decline starting in March 2020, car travel picked up significantly (Sipe, Neil G. (2020). "Cars rule as coronavirus shakes up travel trends in our cities," in *The Conversation*, 20 July 2020, https://bit.ly/3GadUJC).
[275] Department of Industry, Science, Energy and Resources, Australian Government. National Greenhouse Gas Inventory Quarterly Update: December 2020, https://archive.ph/dqRhF.
[276] Statista. "Year-on-year change of weekly flight frequency of global airlines from January 6, 2020 to January 4, 2021, by country," https://bit.ly/3LDABH6.

Counter-balancing these improvements to air quality and (possibly) to natural ecosystems were the damaging environmental impacts of the mountains of masks and additional plastic and other packaging used by shops and restaurants to wrap and ship purchases during lockdowns.

Considering these factors together, I estimate no net "environmental" benefits from lockdowns in Australia. Translating environmental effects like reduced air pollution or increased waste into welfare impacts via their effects on WELLBYs would be a fruitful area of future research but is beyond the scope of this report.

8.5 Estimating the total benefits from lockdowns

Now we can add up the estimated benefits of lockdowns, using the currency of WELLBYs.

8.5.1 *Assumption: Years of life lost from COVID deaths*

In my CBA of UK lockdowns in *The Great Covid Panic*, my co-authors and I assume that the average COVID death involves the loss of three healthy years of life, because most of those who succumbed to COVID were not members of the generally healthy population but suffered from a significant number of co-morbidities.[277]

For Australia, it appears from visual inspection (Figure 3.1) that the median age of those who die from COVID is roughly equivalent to Australians' current life expectancy (as at 4 November 2021, the life expectancy of a baby born in Australia was 81.2 years for males and 85.3 years for females[278]). For earlier cohorts, such as the elderly who have been the vast majority of COVID victims in 2020 and 2021, life expectancy at birth was much lower (e.g., for someone born in 1940 in Australia, life expectancy at birth was around 65.81 years[279]).

[277] Kompaniyets, L. et al (2021). "Underlying Medical Conditions and Severe Illness Among 540,667 Adults Hospitalized With COVID-19, March 2020-March 2021," in *Preventing Chronic Disease*, https://doi.org/10.5888/pcd18.210123.
[278] Australian Bureau of Statistics. Life tables, 4 November 2021, https://bit.ly/3sTigzw.
[279] Statista, https://bit.ly/3LH9gUu, Life expectancy (from birth) in Australia, from 1870 to 2020. Also see: *SuperGuide*. How long you can expect to live, and what it means for your super, https://bit.ly/3wPd4Om.

Nevertheless, I use a more conservative assumption in this report: that the average COVID death involves the loss of five healthy years (i.e., five QALYs) of remaining expected life. This estimate is based on life tables showing the expected QALYs remaining for people with co-morbidities,[280] combined with the observation that about 30% of Australia's COVID deaths have occurred in aged care homes,[281] where on entry a resident is expected to have 1 healthy year of life still to live,[282] with the remaining 70% on average still quite old and with 95% probability suffering from one or more co-morbidities.[283] Assuming a generous 6 years of healthy life remaining on average for the 70% of Australian COVID victims residing outside aged care homes, we arrive at 4.5 years of healthy life remaining per average COVID victim, which I then round up to 5.

One QALY equates to 6 WELLBYs, as explained previously. I therefore assume that each COVID death postponed by lockdowns represents a saving of **30 WELLBYs**.

8.5.2 *Upper limit of the potential benefits from lockdowns*

I use **9,951** deaths as the upper-bound estimate of the number of additional COVID deaths in Australia during 2020 and 2021 without lockdowns.

To this, I add 2% to capture the potential long-COVID suffering that lockdowns might have avoided.

I also add **131** road fatalities and homicides potentially avoided, and allocate to each a loss of 50 healthy years.

I then arrive at the following upper-bound estimate for the total benefit of lockdowns:

---

[280] E.g., Briggs, Andrew (2020). "Estimating QALY losses associated with deaths in hospital (COVID-19)," Research Note, Version 3.0, 22nd April 20, https://bit.ly/3NsoiPl.

[281] Department of Health, Australian Government. Coronavirus (COVID-19) case numbers and statistics, https://bit.ly/3wCN5uA.

[282] Forder, Julien et al (2011). "Length of stay in care homes," Report commissioned by Bupa Care Services, PSSRU Discussion Paper 2769, Canterbury: PSSRU, https://eprints.lse.ac.uk/33895/1/dp2769.pdf.

[283] Liu, Bette et al (2021). "High risk groups for severe COVID-19 in a whole of population cohort in Australia," in *BMC Infectious Diseases*, 21, Article number 685, 16 July 2021, https://bit.ly/3sRxCEp.

9,951 (total COVID deaths averted) x 5 (healthy years lost per COVID death) x 6 (WELLBYs per QALY) x 1.02 (estimate for long COVID) + 131 (non-COVID deaths averted) x 50 (healthy years lost per each such death) x 6 (WELLBYs per QALY) = **343,800** WELLBYs, or **57,300** QALYs, in all.

Dividing this total by 24,[284] we get approximately 14,325 WELLBYs saved per month of stop-start lockdowns, or roughly **560 WELLBYs saved per million per month** (14,325/25.6) during 2020 and 2021.

8.5.3 *How much would society pay to avoid these losses?*

Taking the upper-bound estimate of AU$100,000 as the amount Australian society would be willing to pay to save one QALY, then Australian society would be willing to pay a total of 57,300 (i.e., total QALYs saved) x 100,000 = **AU$5.73 billion** over the course of two years to avoid this magnitude of loss.

In other words, the maximum that Australia would normally be willing to spend to prevent an additional **9,951** COVID deaths *plus* **131** traffic/homicide deaths – even using very conservative assumptions in favour of the government's policies – is around six billion dollars.

In fact, hundreds of billions of dollars have been spent by the Australian government to pursue, enforce, and ameliorate the economic pain of lockdowns. By implication, Australia has paid a minimum of AU$20 million per COVID death possibly averted in 2020 and 2021 with lockdowns. This observation itself, apart from evidence from around the world demonstrating that such costly policies have not even reduced COVID deaths in the medium run, confirms that lockdowns have failed as a policy tool.

The costs of lockdowns that we can compare to the benefits assessed above are enumerated, item by item, in the next four chapters of this report.

---

[284] The precise number of months during which lockdown policies were enacted or threatened is slightly different, since lockdowns started in March 2020 and ended in most parts of Australia before the end of 2021. However, as discussed earlier in the methodological notes, for simplicity I distribute both estimated costs and benefits of the policies across the full years of 2020 and 2021.

8.6 Comment: Assessing the PM's claim that lockdowns have avoided 40,000 deaths

In the lead-up to the election in May 2022, the Prime Minister of Australia is reported to have claimed that 40,000 deaths have been avoided by his "regime" (of lockdowns and border closures).[285] No substantiating evidence was provided, but it is possible that the Prime Minister used estimates from epidemiological models.

Even if Mr Morrison were right and 40,000 COVID deaths had been prevented by lockdowns, that would still bound at **AU\$20 billion** the amount Australia should have paid to pursue the lockdown strategy, using the observation above that Australia is willing to pay at most AU\$100,000 per QALY saved (40,000 x 5 x \$100,000). Spending more than that would divert our limited resources away from other competing and equally deserving priorities.

My estimates above indicate that at most an additional **9,951 COVID deaths** could have been avoided in Australia over the course of two years, not 40,000. Further, as noted above, with over 10,000 reported COVID deaths in Australia during 2022 as at 4 July 2022, a large number of these 9,951 COVID deaths avoided in 2020 and 2021 are likely to have taken place in 2022 – implying that my estimate of 5 years of life saved per COVID death averted in 2020 and 2021 may be too high. (Mr Morrison is not referring to the contribution of traffic fatalities and homicides in his claim, so I exclude these from this discussion.)

As I show in the next chapter, the quantity of human well-being destroyed by Mr Morrison's policies overwhelms the quantity of human well-being that they possibly could have prevented us from losing. Even if lockdowns prevented 9,951 COVID deaths and 131 non-COVID deaths, I estimate that lockdowns have cost Australia around 7,940 additional deaths – mostly in much younger age groups than the average COVID victim – and an enormous range of other harms.

---

[285] *The Guardian* (2022). "Scott Morrison takes credit for saving 40,000 lives from Covid in social media pitch for re-election," 9 April 2022, https://bit.ly/38HctWN.

9. Costs of Australian lockdowns: Overview

The approach taken in *The Great Covid Panic* is one of many ways to think about the costs imposed by lockdown policies. In this chapter I build on the method I used in my PAEC presentation in August 2020, with a number of amendments to expand the analysis and include updated information.

The ensuing analysis, following the tradition of cost-benefit analyses used worldwide to evaluate policies, seeks to quantify the costs of Australia's lockdown policies in different dimensions of life in the short run and the longer run. However, the effects of many government policies – and lockdowns definitely fall into this category – manifest because of changes the policies create in the stocks of the core productive inputs a country can draw on to produce human well-being.

COVID lockdowns have seriously damaged Australia's core stocks of health, human capital more broadly, productive networks, and national wealth. They have reduced trust in government and community cohesion. The impacts of lockdowns as categorised into the various types of costs enumerated below can be seen as ripple effects of these damages to Australia's core productive stocks. In future research on this topic, I hope that the costs of the authoritarianism, loss of good governance, lowered productivity of the state, and loss of institutional trust that lockdowns ushered in will be acknowledged as important underlying elements of the damage they caused, and that attempts will be made to quantify these elements *per se*.

9.1 A typology of costs

Figure 9.1 depicts schematically a classification of the costs of lockdowns and border closures. As detailed in Section 6.1, the costs we are interested in are the residual costs beyond those expected in the counterfactual case, in which some costs would have been incurred even had we used well-targeted and risk-based control measures that were largely voluntary for the general public.

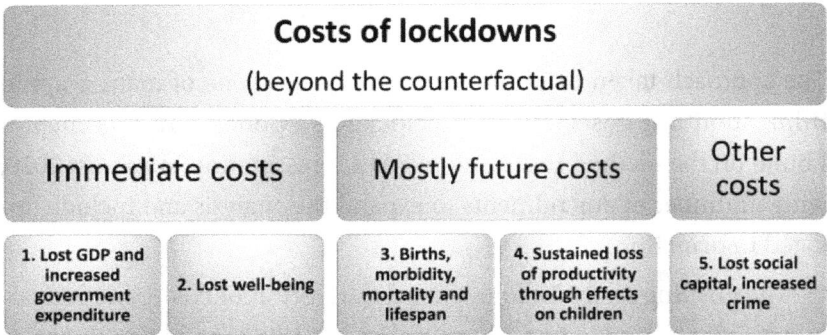

Figure 9.1: A schematic overview of costs considered in this CBA

Given the need to assess each of these cost categories at some length, I split the analysis of these costs of lockdowns into four chapters.

9.2 Websites that are compiling lockdown harms

While I will cite illustrative evidence for various harms in the coming chapters, the illustrations I provide should not be seen as amounting to a comprehensive assessment of these harms. Vast information is now available in the public domain about the harms caused by lockdowns, including in Australia, and this information continues to expand. The following selected websites are among many that are compiling information about lockdown harms from across the world:

> https://collateralglobal.org/physical-health
> https://hereistheevidence.com/covid/
> https://endlockdowns.org/
> http://thepriceofpanic.com/
> https://tomwoods.com/death-by-lockdown/

10.   Immediate costs: (1) Lost GDP and increased expenditure

The world has seen many pandemics in the past, many of which were bigger than the COVID pandemic by orders of magnitude. Yet no prior pandemic, including the Spanish flu, was addressed with policies that caused the general population to suffer economic costs even remotely comparable with those imposed by what the IMF called, in early 2020, the "Great Lockdowns."

On 14 April 2020, the IMF estimated that the cumulative loss to global GDP over 2020 and 2021 from the pandemic crisis could be around 9 trillion dollars.[286]

On 24 January 2021, the International Labour Organisation estimated[287] that "the economic blow from Covid-19 has cost workers around the world $3.7tn in lost earnings, after the pandemic wiped out four times the number of working hours lost in the 2008 financial crisis."

On 21 September 2021, the IMF noted that it "has provided over $118 billion in financing to 87 countries, including 54 low-income countries … [T]he IMF made the largest allocation of Special Drawing Rights in its history – about US$650 billion – injecting additional liquidity to the global economic system." It noted the "sizable fiscal support in advanced economies – with $4.6 trillion of pandemic related measures available in 2021 and beyond."[288]

What is the strictly "economic" price tag in Australia of the unprecedented response to COVID? In this chapter I look at the immediate economic costs of lockdowns, which I then convert into hu-

---

[286] Gopinath, Gita (2020). "The Great Lockdown: Worst Economic Downturn Since the Great Depression," IMF blogs, 14 April 2020, https://bit.ly/3wCxRWf.

[287] *The Guardian* (2021). "Covid-19 has cost global workers $3.7tn in lost earnings, says ILO," 25 January 2021, https://bit.ly/3wIZ4FF.

[288] Sayeh, Antoinette M. (2021). "A New Agenda for Macro Stability," International Monetary Fund, 21 September 2021, https://bit.ly/3MG0nfm.

man well-being costs for the purpose of subsequent comparisons and calculations.

10.1 Illustrative economic costs

A wide range of economic harms were caused by lockdowns. Illustratively:

Impact on entrepreneurs and businesses

- Loss of business or employment due not being able to meet costs, loss of clients, and restrictions, with small business particularly impacted.

- Businesses that will never be able to recover and re-establish, meaning broken productive chains.

- Disruption to transportation, logistics, and production leading to disrupted supply chains.

- Disheartened entrepreneurs and workers, leading to productivity losses.

Increased poverty and disadvantage

- Increased homelessness due to debt pressures on credit cards, personal loans, mortgages and/or rent repayments.

- Increased numbers of people permanently dropping out of the labour force.

- Increased poverty leading to reduced capacity to manage physical and mental health; increased dependence on the state, public housing, income support, and the health system.

- Increased inequality, with those who worked secure jobs from home benefiting while many others lost.

- Movement "off grid" of people who have decided it is no longer worthwhile to engage in society.

- Fewer employment opportunities, particularly for young people, and reduced training; increased uptake of drug use and other poor habits that may persist.

Largely futile activity that reduced productivity

- Productive resources wasted in often futile "contact tracing" and QR code checking.
- Increased transaction costs required to obtain goods and services; interstate postage delays.

Other impacts on productivity

- Dramatically reduced skilled immigration leading to an associated skills shortage.
- Increased unemployment, underemployment, and poor-quality job-employee matching.
- Loss of experienced staff and the early retirement of those unable to find new jobs.

Sectoral impacts

- Short- and longer-term financial impacts on education institutions due to lack of international student income.
- Loss of domestic and international tourism revenue.
- Loss of revenue and careers in the arts and entertainment industries.

Impact on public finances

- Loss of tax revenue, carrying implications for the provision of public goods today (e.g., for maintenance of public infrastructure) and in the future.
- Large fiscal outlays contributing to medium-run inflation risk and leading to crippling government debt left to future generations.

10.2 Some evidence for the economic costs of lockdowns

The Harvard School of Public Health reported on 23 June 2021 that in Africa, COVID-19 restrictions impacted food systems, resulting in reported price increases for grains, pulses (lentils, chickpeas, and beans), fruits, vegetables, and animal-source foods, and decreased consumption of diverse and quality diets.[289]

---

[289] https://www.eurekalert.org/news-releases/913486.

It was reported on 8 December 2020 by Bloomberg about the USA that "[m]ore than 110,000 restaurants have closed permanently or long-term across the country as the industry grapples with the devastating impact of the Covid-19 pandemic. ...'more than 500,000 restaurants of every business type – franchise, chain and independent – are in an economic free fall."[290]

An analysis of the performance of Australia's retail sector's shows that a huge shock (in some cases positive) went through the sector in 2020 and continued in 2021. Many smaller retail stores would not have been able to cope with this huge change in demand and will have permanently shut down.

10.3 Estimating the economic costs

To estimate the immediate economic costs of lockdowns, I focus on two categories:

   a) Lost production (lost GDP)

   b) Increased transfers and stimulus (increased government debt)

10.3.1 *Lost production (lost GDP)*

The goal of this estimation effort is to identify only the loss of production which is over and above the production that would have been lost had Australia followed approximately the COVID policies of Sweden, a country with no lockdowns that serves as a counterfactual. To do this, adjustments must be made to Sweden's observed outcomes to account for differences in the economic structure of the two countries.

Australia's GDP shrank 7% in the April-to-June 2020 quarter compared with the previous three months.[291,292] In comparison,

---

[290] *Mercury News* (2020). "U.S. restaurant closings top 110,000 with industry in 'free fall," 8 December 2020, https://bit.ly/3PEe8Ng.

[291] Department of Mines, Industry Regulation and Safety, Government of Western Australia, "WA resources sector's biggest year ever powering nation through COVID," 11 October 2021, https://bit.ly/3NprD1w.

[292] *BBC News* (2020). "Australia in first recession for nearly 30 years," 2 September 2020, https://bit.ly/3PAimpo.

in Sweden, in "the second quarter as a whole, GDP grew by 0.9 percent, seasonally adjusted and compared with the previous quarter."[293] By the end of the year, however, GDP in Sweden had shrunk by 2.8%[294] even as Australia's had only shrunk by 0.3%.[295] (To gauge both nations' performance I use World Bank data, to maximise comparability).

This leads to the result that Sweden seems to have ended up with a worse impact on production than Australia. However, this headline result hides important methodological and structural differences that I detail below.

a) *Major pandemic transfer payments were included in Australia's GDP.* In the case of Australia, the ABS decided to include JobKeeper as part of GDP, unlike the approach it takes for other transfers:

> JobKeeper payments will provide an estimated $70 billion of support from the Australian Government to eligible employers. The payments will be made by the Australian Taxation Office directly to eligible employers who will be directly responsible for ensuring that eligible employees receive a wage of at least $1,500 per fortnight for a maximum period of six months commencing on 30 March 2020.[296]

JobKeeper paid out AU$89bn and ended in March 2021.[297] Including JobKeeper payments in GDP is arguably misleading, since production did not occur in most cases: organisations had their doors closed and output was significantly impacted, which was the rationale for the government payments. Even were JobKeeper to be included, the fact that JobKeeper payments were transfers made by taxpayers, rather than prices paid within markets, requires them to be recorded differently. Correctly attributing JobKeeper would both

---

[293] Statistics Sweden (2021). "GDP indicator: Continued growth in June 2021," 29 July 2021, https://bit.ly/3LDC5RG.
[294] World Bank, GDP growth (annual %) – Sweden, https://bit.ly/3SbheKb.
[295] World Bank, GDP growth (annual %) – Australia, https://bit.ly/3bkV87o.
[296] Australian Bureau of Statistics (2020). Economic measurement during COVID-19: Selected issues in the Economic Accounts, 18 May 2020, https://bit.ly/3yOt7OV.
[297] *The Guardian* (2021). "The 2021 federal budget reveals huge $311bn cost of Covid to Australian economy," 11 May 2021, https://bit.ly/3wBMQ2E.

reduce GDP and inflate transfers. $89 billion is around 6% of Australia's GDP, meaning the impact of treating JobKeeper as a production equivalent rather than as a transfer payment is not negligible.

b) *Structure of the economy*: Australia had radically different drivers of GDP in 2020 and 2021 compared to Sweden. Mining constitutes only 1.3% of Sweden's GDP but over 10.4% of Australia's. This matters because during the pandemic, production dropped in most countries and China took up more of the global production load, leading to a boom in the import of minerals into China from Australia, which in turn significantly boosted Australia's GDP. Illustratively, "Minerals and petroleum sales in WA grew by $38 billion to $210 billion from 2019-20 to 2020-21."[298]

Australia also produces high-end products such as software (though few manufactured goods). During the pandemic, high-end software production also kept pace in Australia since it was a natural complement to the trend of working from home. Except for tourism and education, overall exports from Australia also saw continued strong growth. For example, in 2021 it was reported that "[t]he value of Australia's exports to China has jumped 24% from a year ago, to reach over $180 billion Australian dollars ($135 billion) as of the latest August data."[299]

For reasons like these, a direct GDP comparison between Australia and Sweden is fraught. Further, sector-specific losses felt in Australian service industries like education, hospitality, tourism, and retail were barely evident in counterpart Swedish industries.

As a conservative guess, I assume for this report that Australia suffered a production loss equivalent to 0.5% of its GDP during both 2020 and 2021 beyond what it would have seen under a counterfactual covid policy approach like Sweden's. This estimate in-

---

[298] Media statement dated 10 October 2021 by the West Australian government: "WA resources sector's biggest year ever powering nation through COVID," https://archive.ph/5yw1I.

[299] CNBC News (2021). "Australia's exports to China are jumping despite their trade fight," 27 October 2021, https://bit.ly/3wJeMR5.

cludes the awareness that lockdowns mainly affected Victoria and NSW, even though other states did have significant reductions in international tourism and education. Further, the increase in mining production (which benefits relatively few workers) does not offset the permanent loss of production in other higher-employment sectors. It can be argued that an estimated production loss of 0.5% of GDP is conservative.

A loss of 0.5% of GDP means Australia lost about $7.5 billion dollars' worth of production per year in each of the two years of lockdowns.

10.3.2 *Increased government expenditure*

In addition to lost production, we need to take account of the huge increase in expenditure by the government during 2020 and 2021. Sweden did not require a major stimulus since it did not so significantly cripple its own economy. The impact on health care costs was probably similar in both countries, even as elective surgeries were not as disrupted in Sweden as in Australia.

In September 2020, the Institute of Public Affairs observed that the expenditures made as part of the attempt to contain COVID amounted to more than the total usually spent per year on most major government expenditure line items. As Adam Creighton reported, "[f]rom June this year to the middle of 2022, the "elimination strategy" being pursued by state and federal governments will cost $319bn, equivalent to 23 per cent of GDP, according to the report, Medical Capacity: An Alternative to Lockdowns."[300]

To estimate the value of increased expenditure in 2020 and 2021, I look at the increase in deficit financing by Australia relative to recent years. The combined Federal, state and local government deficit funding during 2020-21 was $263 billion (12.8 per cent of GDP). In 2021-22, it is projected to be $193 billion (9 per cent of GDP).[301]

---

[300] Creighton, Adam (2020). "Coronavirus: Elimination strategy 'will cost us $319bn,'" in *The Australian*, 29 September 2020, https://bit.ly/2ELCrcP.
[301] Mizen, Ronald et al (2021). "Total Australian state and federal government debt to double to $2trn," in *Financial Review*, 23 June 2021, https://bit.ly/38KeHVp.

In comparison, the 2017 federal budget forecast a deficit of AU$29.3 billion, or 1.6% of GDP. The 2018 budget forecast a deficit of AU$18.2 billion.[302] If we generously assume that without COVID, the fiscal deficit for all Australian governments in 2020 and 2021 would have been $50 billion in each year, and therefore reduce the actual fiscal deficits of Australia in 2020-21 and 2021-22 ($456 billion) by AU$100 billion, we recover AU$356 billion as the estimate of the net additional cost to Australia's taxpayers of living through COVID.

Aum et al (2020) estimate that around one-half of all job losses in the UK and the US can be attributed to lockdowns.[303] Applying this bifurcation of economic damage to the sphere of government fiscal outlays during COVID, I assume that half of the estimated additional expenditure of AU$356 billion would have been spent by the government even if it had followed largely voluntary policies to combat COVID rather than lockdowns and border closures. This then yields an estimate of AU$178 billion as the additional financial cost to taxpayers that can be attributed directly to lockdown policies in 2020 and 2021.

10.3.3 *Increased inequality, and inflation impacts on the poor*

There is significant evidence from across the world that lockdown policies have disproportionately harmed the poor. In addition, there is emerging evidence that the supply bottlenecks created by the lockdowns and border closures have raised prices of a wide range of commodities and inputs for manufactured goods.[304] This has led to an erratic global economic recovery and threatens to lower the relative standard of living of the poor even further.

In the absence of sufficient data at this stage, I will ignore the immediate economic effects of lockdowns on inequality, but the harm of increased inequality as well as the impacts of inflation which has emerged globally in 2022 should be included in future estimates of

---

[302] *Wikipedia*. Australian government debt, 29 April 2022, https://bit.ly/3wCfiBB.

[303] Aum, Sangmin et al (2020). "Doesn't Need Lockdowns to Destroy Jobs: The Effect of Local Outbreaks in Korea," CEPR Discussion Paper 14822, https://archive.ph/OzmiS.

[304] See, indicatively, "Chart Pack, Australian Inflation," 6 July 2022, Reserve Bank of Australia, https://archive.ph/rK9kD.

the costs of lockdowns. These issues are even more important in developing countries that have weak social safety nets. For instance, on 26 September 2020, the Economist magazine reported the World Bank's research estimating that due to the lockdowns the number of extremely poor people (those who earn less than US$1.90 a day) would rise by 70 to 100 million in that year.[305] A 28 October 2020 Indian Express article notes: "The new urban poor in Mumbai: Salaries gone, pawning gold to pay school fees, NGO meals, rents unpaid."[306]

10.3.4 *Economic cost of lockdowns in WELLBYs*

We can now convert the estimate of conventional economic losses to Australia created by COVID lockdowns and related policies into a monthly figure in the currency of WELLBYs.

Dividing the AU$178 billion increase in the fiscal deficit by the 24 months in 2020 and 2021 yields a monthly cost of AU$7.42 billion.[307] Adding to this AU$7.5 billion/12 = AU$0.625 billion as the monthly cost of lost production yields a total of AU$8.045 billon per month of conventional economic loss.

How much welfare loss does this represent? Since lockdowns were billed as a form of public health policy, we can view this question as asking for an "exchange rate" between dollars and welfare based on how much welfare our expenditures on public health policies and programs normally buy. Some estimates of how much welfare (denominated in QALYs) is gained from Australia's health expenditure

---

[305] *The Economist* (2020). "Covid-19 has reversed years of gains in the war on poverty," 26 September 2020, https://archive.ph/aOe2F.

[306] *The Indian Express*. "The new urban poor in Mumbai: Salaries gone, pawning gold to pay school fees, NGO meals, rents unpaid," 28 October 2020, https://archive.ph/a3iqT.

[307] As discussed earlier in the methodological notes, a more exact approach would recognise that lockdowns began only at the end of March 2020, and hence would split costs like this one up into monthly segments separately by year, i.e., dividing annual totals by 9 to recover 2020 monthly costs and by an appropriate figure (perhaps 10 or 11) to recover 2021 monthly costs. Apart from being more complex, this would increase the monthly cost estimates. I aim to assess the costs of Australia's COVID response both approximately and conservatively, while preserving clarity, and have opted to use the simpler calculation that treats all months in 2020 and 2021 as "stop-start lockdown" months for these reasons. Refining these estimates by adjusting this aspect of the analysis is a task I expect governments and researchers to undertake in future.

are extracted from several analyses below to help us answer this question.

- "In Australia, public summaries for each assessed pharmaceutical are published. Recent documents suggest new drugs are generally recommended if their expected incremental cost per QALY is somewhere between $45,000 and $75,000" (2015).[308]

- "a gain of 1 QALY is expected for every additional A$28 033 of government expenditure on health" (2018).[309]

- "For Australia, an intervention that costs between A$37 000 to A$112 000/QALY is regarded as being cost effective" (2006).[310]

These studies suggest a range of health expenditure between $28,000 and $112,000 in current dollars to purchase one QALY of health. I take a mid-to-high-range estimate in order to be generous to lockdowns, and assume that public health expenditure of $100,000 buys one QALY. This yields an equivalence of the economic cost of the public health policy of lockdowns to a loss of 80,450 QALYs per month, and therefore (multiplying QALYs by 6) 482,700 WELLBYs per month assuming the gains purchased were in the form of life-years saved.

---

[308] Karnon, Jonathan et al (2015). "New cancer drugs are very expensive – here's how we work out value for our money," in *The Conversation*, 8 September 2015, https://bit.ly/3887PRi.

[309] Edney, Laura et al (2018), "Are the benefits of new health services greater than their opportunity costs?" in *Australian Health Review*, 43(5) 508-510, https://archive.ph/pFugS.

[310] https://www.ncbi.nlm.nih.gov/pmc/articles/PMC1856946/, Taylor, H.M. et al (2006), "The economic impact and cost of visual impairment in Australia," *Br J Ophthalmol.* 2006 Mar; 90(3): 272–275.

11. Immediate costs: (2) Lost well-being

The loss of happiness because of lockdowns, due for example to loneliness and impacts on relationships from enforced social isolation, is an important aspect of the cost of COVID lockdowns that was nearly completely ignored by Australia's policy-makers in 2020 and 2021.

11.1 Illustrative mental harms and low-level violence

Illustrative mental harms include mental stress, depression and anxiety from:

- loneliness (about forty per cent of Australians live in one-person households. Many of these people were subject to effective solitary confinement for weeks or months at a time during which they did not see a real human face in person due to mandatory masking)

- loneliness of the elderly in care homes that banned visitors (although some impacts in this area would likely have occurred under less extreme COVID policies, such as targeted protection for the elderly)

- mental suffering of labouring mothers who were not allowed support persons at the time of birth in hospitals, and interference with normal maternal/paternal/infant bonding

- loss of contact with friends and family leading to sadness and strained relations

- cancellation/postponement/alteration of weddings, funerals, and other milestone event celebrations, with related emotional toll

- broken family ties due to extended separations; breakdown of childhood bonds created with friends and extended family

- impact on mental health and relationships (including relationship breakdown in some cases) of unemployment, concerns about financial and health security, anxiety about the future, and overall stress

The results of some of these mental harms were expressed in physical form, e.g.:

- increased risk of domestic violence
- suicidal thoughts or tendency for self-harm
- increased abuse of drugs and alcohol

11.2 A snapshot of the evidence

Evidence on the mental harms caused by lockdowns will one day fill many books. I provide merely a snapshot below.

11.2.1 *Australian evidence*

On 10 July 2020, it was reported that:

> More and more Victorians in crisis are reaching out to Lifeline Australia's suicide prevention and crisis support services. In the past week alone, Lifeline Australia has noted a 22 per cent spike in calls originating from Victoria.[311]

A report to the Victorian Parliament by a Parliamentary Committee in July 2020 noted anecdotal reports about the increase in family violence:

> In the early stages of the COVID-19 pandemic, the Victorian Government responded to a concern about a spike in family violence by providing funding to the sector and initiating a pro-active policing campaign, Operation Ribbon. However, data is not yet available to determine whether these activities were successful in limiting family violence. During the hearings stakeholders provided anecdotal evidence to suggest that the rate and type of violence used during the pandemic had changed and possibly escalated. In addition, the COVID-19 pandemic created real and perceived barriers to service access for victim survivors, while there have been notable gendered impacts of the pandemic.[312]

---

[311] *Bendigo Advertiser* (2020). "Lifeline reports 22 per cent spike in Victorian calls as the COVID-19 pandemic worsens," 10 July 2022, https://archive.ph/gIJ2C.

[312] PAEC, *Inquiry into the Victorian Government's response to the COVID-19 pandemic - Interim report*, July 2020, https://bit.ly/389uf4N.

The Australian National University is reported to have found that 20% of respondents in a survey were drinking more alcohol since the start of lockdowns.[313]

It was reported in *ABC News* on 8 August 2020 that: "Department of Health and Human Services data shows Victoria has recorded a 33 per cent rise in children presenting to hospital with self-harm injuries over the past six weeks, compared to a year earlier."[314]

On 10 August 2020 it was reported that: "In response to the increasing number of people having a hard time coping with the pandemic, the Victorian government yesterday announced an additional A$59.7 million in funding for mental health services."[315]

On 11 September 2020 the Chief Health Officer of Victoria[316] admitted to the significant impact on the well-being of Victorians from "the measures" (lockdowns) to "slow the spread of coronavirus" – but did not quantify or assess the harms or commit to a process to do so:

> 81. I acknowledge the measures taken to slow the spread of coronavirus will have a significant impact on the well-being of Victorians, especially those who are living or parenting alone, as well as those who have mental health conditions or other complex needs.
>
> 82. While there has been evidence of the strong resilience of the Victorian community during the state of emergency (for example, a Coroner's Court of Victoria report on 27 August 2020 found that the number of suicide fatalities remained consistent at 466 this year compared to 468 from last year), there is significant evidence of the community's distress due to the significant limits on social movement and interaction

---

[313] *ABC News* (2020). "Why women were more likely to drink alcohol than men during the coronavirus lockdown," 9 June 2020, https://archive.ph/h9HC3.

[314] Clayton, Rachel (2020). "Statistics show increase in children presenting to hospitals after self-harming," in *ABC News*, 8 August 2020, https://bit.ly/3NtPn4D.

[315] Maylea, Chris (2020). "The Victorian government has allocated $60 million to mental health. But who gets the money?" in *The Conversation*, 10 August 2020, https://bit.ly/3sRuBUO.

[316] State of Victoria: Advice relating to Declaration of Extension to State of Emergency, from Chief Health Officer Advice to Minister for Health, 11 September 2020, https://bit.ly/389686j – extracted from a Parliamentary document.

(such as a 40% increase in calls to Lifeline when restrictions were strengthened in August 2020).

It was reported on 16 September 2020 that:

> Nurses sent in to help Melbourne's coronavirus-ravaged aged care facilities say they are gravely concerned for residents – even those without COVID-19 infections – who have been stuck in "solitary confinement" for months. One resident has even refused to eat and drink because she can't see her family or leave her room.[317]

On 14 October 2020, The Australian reported that:

> More than a million Australians have sought mental health treatment during the COVID-19 pandemic, while ongoing lockdowns in Victoria have sparked a social crisis, with a 30 per cent rise in cases in the past four weeks.
>
> The first official data revealing the depth of the mental health disaster in Victoria since the second wave outbreak reveals access to some crisis services has risen by up to 67 per cent in the space of four weeks.
>
> Demand for children's mental health has also skyrocketed in Victoria, with access to services jumping more than 30 per cent since September.
>
> [I]n September and October, 350,884 Victorians sought access to Medicare-funded GPs, psychiatrists, psychologists and counselling treatments. This was a 31 per cent increase on the same period last year and three times higher than the national average.
>
> According to the data, there were 3702 calls to the Kids Helpline by Victorians, a 61 per cent increase in just four weeks.
>
> Access to Beyond Blue services in Victoria was 77 per cent higher than the rest of the country. The total number of contacts to the mental health organisation was 6472 over the same four weeks – a 67 per cent increase on the same time last year – compared with a 27 per cent increase in NSW and 8 per cent nationally.

---

[317] *ABC News* (2020). "Aged care residents giving up due to COVID-19 and isolation, nurses fear," 15 September 2020, https://bit.ly/3yRb4HI.

Victorian use of Lifeline services was 16 per cent higher than the rest of the country and Kids Helpline 24 per cent higher. Victoria's own data showed a 33 per cent spike in "child and youth contacts in community mental health services for eating disorders."[318]

It was reported on 15 October 2020 that according to Victoria's Department of Health and Human Services, the number of people presenting to emergency departments for treatment for self-harm and suicidal ideation increased 5.7 per cent in 2020 compared with the same period in the previous year. For young people aged 17 and under, the rate had risen 31.3 per cent, as of September 25, when compared with the previous year.[319]

On 28 August 2021 a news report noted that "Teen mental health hospitalizations [rose] by 57% during lockdowns in Victoria."[320]

A 1 October 2021 paper reported on surveys in April and in July/August 2020 in Australia finding that "The most severe COVID-19 restrictions are associated with near double the population prevalence of moderate to severe depressive and generalised anxiety symptoms."[321]

While episodes of enforced non-employment in Australia were relatively short except in Victoria, there are extremely harmful health consequences of wanting to work but being unable to – including morbidity and mortality. There is a proven statistical link between unemployment and health outcomes.

According to one study a 1 percent increase in the unemployment rate will be associated with 37,000 deaths [includ-

[318] Benson, Simon (2020). "Mental health crisis: One million 'lost' in coronavirus lockdown," in *The Australian*, 14 October 2020, https://bit.ly/3wCteeN.

[319] Varga, Remy (2020). "Coronavirus: Number of suicide attempts surges during lockdown," in *The Australian*, 15 October 2020, https://bit.ly/3MR5Tvu.

[320] *RT.com* (2021). "Teen mental health hospitalizations rise by 57% during lockdowns in Victoria – state report," 28 August 2021, https://bit.ly/3Nrdl0s.

[321] https://www.ncbi.nlm.nih.gov/pmc/articles/PMC8264352/, Fisher, Jane et al (2021). "Quantifying the mental health burden of the most severe covid-19 restrictions: A natural experiment," in *J Affect Disord*, 2021 Oct 1; 293: 406–414. 2 July 2021 doi: 10.1016/j.jad.2021.06.060.

ing 20,000 heart attacks], 920 suicides, 650 homicides, 4,000 state mental hospital admissions and 3,300 state prison admissions.[322]

On 11 January 2022 it was reported that "[s]tress has emerged as a key driver increasing alcohol intake during COVID-19, consistent with the 'self-medication hypothesis' for substance use...One of Australia's leading bank institutions has reported a sustained increase in spending on alcohol by both low- and higher-income households between May 2020 to February 2021 compared with the previous year... Twenty per cent of respondents to a 2020 poll by Australian National University (ANU) also reported increased alcohol use... The Australian Drug Foundation found that 29% of parents increased their drinking, with 14% reporting drinking daily... Prior to the pandemic, the cost of alcohol-related harms to Australia was estimated at $67 billion, but the current trends associated with CO-VID-19 suggest this cost is likely to be higher still."[323]

There are reports of changes in drug use in Australia during the pandemic, with indications of stress or depression as the causes.[324] The precise magnitude of the durability of any such changes and their longer-term health impacts will take time to determine.

There were 3,192 suicides reported in Australia in 2018, 3,318 in 2019 and 3,139 in 2020.[325] When we examine the age-standardised suicide rate (per 100,000) over time, we find no strong deviation from trend (Figure 11.1).

---

[322] Crudele, John (2020), "Is unemployment really as deadly as coronavirus?" in *New York Post*, 20 April 2020, https://bit.ly/3yTtXK9.

[323] *NewsGP*. "Has COVID-19 changed Australia's alcohol consumption?" 11 January 2022, https://archive.ph/oitpQ.

[324] *ABC News*. "Survey reveals major shift in Australian drug use during coronavirus pandemic," 7 November 2020, https://archive.ph/MApJ9.

[325] Australian Institute of Health and Welfare, Data tables: 2020 National Mortality Database – Suicide (ICD-10 X60–X84, Y87.0) at https://bit.ly/3wBjznu.

Age-standardised suicide rate (per 100,000), Australia, 2010-2020

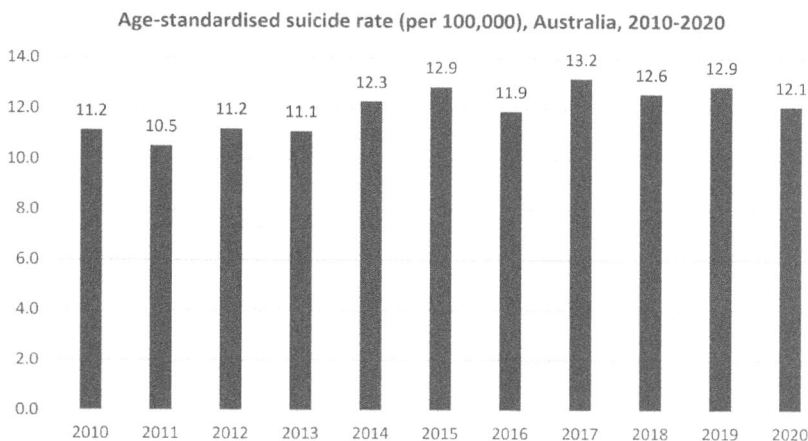

Figure 11.1: Age-standardised suicide rate (per 100,000), Australia, 2010-2020 (Source: AIHW[326])

While the number of reported suicides in Australia did not increase in 2020, in some other countries, like India, they did. For instance, on 31 October 2021 the National Crime Records Bureau of India released data to show that 11,396 children died by suicide in 2020, an 18 per cent rise from 9,613 such deaths in 2019.[327]

11.2.2 Evidence from other countries

Professor Ellen Townsend of the Self-Harm Research Group at the University of Nottingham made a submission to the UK Parliament on 10 January 2021 in which she noted that "high quality prospective data indicates that lockdown in March increased the number of young people with diagnosable mental health problems – 1 in 6 in 2020 as compared to 1 in 9 in 2017."[328]

It was reported on 30 August 2020 that in the UK, domestic-abuse hotline calls were up over 60%. Drug abuse and alcoholism were also up.[329]

---

[326] *Ibid.* These data may be revised in future.
[327] *NDTV* (2021). "31 Children Died By Suicide Every Day In India In 2020," 31 October 2021, https://bit.ly/3yPiBXG.
[328] Written evidence from Professor Ellen Townsend (CIL0977), UK Parliament, https://bit.ly/3wHIbv8.
[329] Carter, Michael P. (2020). "Counting the Cost of U.K., U.S. Lockdowns," in Letters, *Wall Street Journal*, 30 August 2020, https://on.wsj.com/3kQexvT.

It was reported by the organisation Endlockdowns that:

> Since lockdowns began, numerous studies have already captured a surge in the number of people moving towards suicide. In a survey of university students in Greece, suicidal thoughts had increased 8-fold compared to pre-lockdown. According to the CEO of the Canadian Mental Health Association, calls to its hotlines have increased 50-60%. A hospital trust in the UK reported seeing as many suicide attempts in the first few weeks of lockdown as it saw in all of 2019.[330]

An article on 25 October 2020 described the devastating effects of lockdowns on mental health in Argentina:[331]

> Three out of four people, or seventy-five percent, now have sleep problems in Buenos Aires, while one in two have decided to stop daily activities...
>
> "Having more than 200 days without pleasant stimuli, such as social meetings, trips or outings affected my motivation...even more so knowing that the economic situation in my context is terrifying," said Azul Weimann, who is in the third year of studying to be a nutritionist and now has sleeping problems and an eating disorder.
>
> Another resident, a woman named Julieta who works nine hours a day from home, said she has had anxiety attacks and is now undergoing therapy.

Endlockdowns (which provides detailed references) has reported that:

> The psychological harms of social isolation often manifest themselves as depression. Many studies have captured a sharp rise in depression and anxiety since lockdowns began. According to one study, a third of Americans are now displaying clinical-level depression. A Greek study discovered a major increase in mental health issues among university students: 42.5% for anxiety, 74.3% for depression, and

---

[330] *Lockdown Resistance*. Suicide, https://bit.ly/3LzQ3UJ.
[331] SamadiMD (website of David Samadi), "Psychological Trauma Mounting in Argentina – Lockdowns Do Not Discriminate," 25 October 2020, https://bit.ly/3LD9xry.

a 63.3% increase in suicidal thoughts. A common finding across lockdown mental health surveys around the world is that approximately 25% of people are now experiencing severe mental distress.[332]

Further, it notes that:

A survey by UK's Office for National Statistics found that 20% of people that drink alcohol daily have increased their consumption. The Canadian Centre of Substance Abuse and Addiction discovered that 25% of people aged 35 to 54 have been drinking more.[333]

And that:

New research from the University of Bristol has found that loneliness has multiple effects on smoking – it leads to the commencement of smoking, an increase in the number of cigarettes smoked per day in existing smokers, and makes it less likely to quit smoking. These effects are greater in longer periods of social isolation according to the research team. Probably the most surprising finding of the study was that being socially isolated results in many people taking up smoking for the first time, flying in the face of the traditional view that people only start smoking due to peer pressure.[334]

An 11 April 2022 study in the USA found that "[s]moking increased in those trying to quit during COVID-19."[335]

Philipp Bagus et al pointed out on 3 February 2021 that:[336]

Especially lockdowns have contributed to a surge in anxiety and stress, which are important ingredients for the development of mass hysteria ... In a survey conducted in the US

---

[332] *Lockdown Resistance*. Isolation, https://bit.ly/3wyHPrH.
[333] *Lockdown Resistance*. Substance Use, https://bit.ly/39MwdZ5.
[334] *Lockdown Resistance*. Smoking, https://bit.ly/3PClKjn.
[335] *Science Daily*. "Smoking increased in those trying to quit during COVID-19, study shows," 11 April 2022, https://www.sciencedaily.com/releases/2022/04/220411101404.htm.
[336] Bagus, Philipp et al (2021). "COVID-19 and the Political Economy of Mass Hysteria," in *International Journal of Environmental Research and Public Health* 2021, 18(4), 1376; https://doi.org/10.3390/ijerph18041376.

from 24 to 30 June, 40.9% of participants reported at least one adverse mental health condition, and 10.7% reported to have considered suicide seriously in the last 30 days. Additionally, the frequency of alcohol consumption during lockdowns increased 14% in the US.

An 18 May 2021 report noted the findings of an article published in the International Journal of Mental Health Nursing, that the COVID-19 pandemic presents the "perfect storm" for family violence, where a set of rare circumstances have combined to aggravate intimate partner violence, domestic abuse, domestic violence, and child abuse.[337]

A 9 June 2021 news report noted that Kids Helpline data revealed that "attempted suicide rates among Victorian teenagers [soared] by 184 per cent in [the previous] six months."[338]

A 26 August 2021 BBC report on the Northern Ireland Commissioner for Children and Young People study of the well-being of young people notes:

> Many children and young people said they felt "lonely and trapped" during lockdowns and due to restrictions.
>
> "It is clear from the children and young people with whom we engaged through surveys and focus groups how important friendships and developing relationships are throughout childhood and into the teenage years, and how deeply they have felt the restrictions on their social interactions," the report said.
>
> "The research data shows that the decline in play, recreational and leisure activities has had a devastating impact on many children's physical health and emotional well-being."[339]

---

[337] *EurekaAlert*. "COVID-19 pandemic has created the "perfect storm" for family violence," 19 May 2021, https://bit.ly/3wHkEKE.

[338] *News.com.au* (2021). "Attempted suicide rates among Victorian teenagers soar by 184 per cent in past six months, Kids Helpline reveals," 9 June 2021, https://bit.ly/3sQbjim.

[339] *BBC News* (2021). "Covid-19: Pandemic had severe impact on young people, says report," 26 August 2021, https://bit.ly/3wCtVop.

An extensive list of further examples of mental health harms is provided at https://archive.ph/5OCVP, mainly from the EurekAlert website of the research-dissemination arm of the American Association for the Advancement of Science, the world's largest general scientific society with over 120,000 members that publishes the well-known scientific journal Science.

11.3 Measuring the immediate harms to well-being

As discussed previously, in this report I use overall life satisfaction as the primary proxy for human well-being.

What does this measure look like in normal times, and what happened to it during lockdowns?

The OECD[340] finds that when asked to rate their general satisfaction with life on a scale from 0 to 10, Australians on average selected 7.3 and the British people on average 6.8, both of which are higher than the OECD average response of 6.5.

11.3.1 *UK Life Satisfaction surveys*

The UK Office for National Statistics conducts two surveys[341] on life satisfaction using different data collection methods: the Annual Population Survey (APS) that relies on telephone interviews, and the Opinions and Lifestyle Survey (abbreviated 'OPN') that uses online self-completion.

Figure 11.2 reproduces portions from Figures 1 and 2 in the 4 February 2021 ONS survey report depicting the trajectory of life satisfaction across different stages of the pandemic based on data from these two different surveys.

---

[340] OECD Better Life Index. Life Satisfaction, https://bit.ly/3BlxCSr.
[341] Office for National Statistics. "Data collection changes due to the pandemic and their impact on estimating personal well-being," 4 February 2021, https://bit.ly/3wDFH27.

Annual Population Survey

Overall, how **satisfied** are you with your life nowadays?

Opinions and Lifestyle Survey

Overall, how **satisfied** are you with your life nowadays?

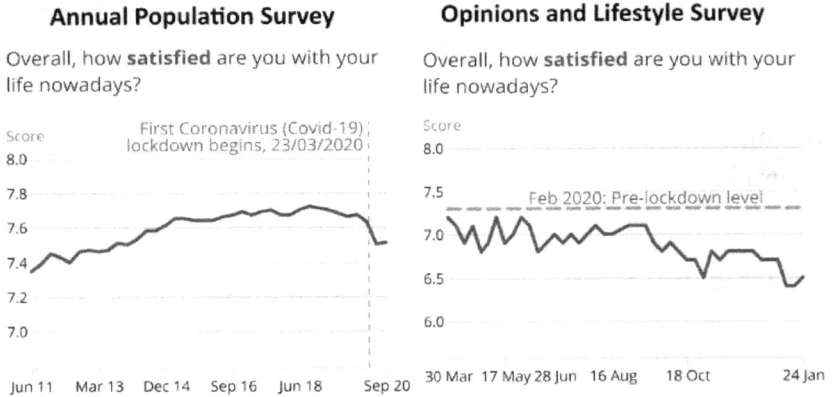

Figure 11.2: The measurement of life satisfaction using two different surveys by the ONS in the UK

Note: The x-axis for the APS graph (from Figure 1 of the ONS report) depicts quarterly snapshots from April 2011 to September 2020. The x-axis for the OPN graph (taken from Figure 2 of the ONS report) is for the eight months of 2020-2021 during which the survey was conducted.

The APS survey suggests that life satisfaction was gently increasing in the UK until it dropped steeply, by around 0.1 points (from 7.6 to 7.5) on the typical 0-to-10-point scale, over the first six months of lockdowns.[342] The OPN survey shows an even more dramatic drop of over 0.5 points between March 2020 and January 2021.

Normally I would select the more conservative of these results (i.e., the lower figure) as an estimate of the well-being costs of the UK lockdowns, but in this case there is an important methodological concern. After March 2020, the methodology for the APS changed significantly, with face-to-face interaction replaced with telephone interviews. This led to a shift in sample composition, including a notable decrease in the proportion of respondents who live in rented accommodation. While housing tenure was added to the weighting process in an attempt to mitigate the potential non-response bias caused by this operational change, I consider the OPN survey to be a more reliable data source for this question as its methodology did not change during the pandemic.

---

[342] Clark, A. E., Flèche, S., Layard, R., Powdthavee, N., & Ward, G. (2018). *The Origins of Happiness: The Science of Well-Being Over the Life Course*, NJ: Princeton University Press.

11.3.2 *Australian life satisfaction survey: HILDA*

The Household, Income and Labour Dynamics in Australia (HIL-DA) survey run by the University of Melbourne follows the lives of more than 17,000 Australians each year. Arguably Australia's best longitudinal social scientific survey, HILDA offers a time series since 2001 and includes a number of questions related to well-being, including this one: "All things considered, how satisfied are you with your life overall?" Responses range from 0 to 10. The higher this score, the more satisfied a person is with his or her life as a whole.

The 15th Annual Statistical Report of the HILDA Survey,[343] published on 20 November 2020, contains the responses to this question through 2018. The mean life satisfaction for all persons and by sex over the years has shown remarkable stability. The well-being measure has remained largely within the narrow band of 7.85 and 7.95 since 2012.

The 16th HILDA report of 2021 has no comparable chart, nor is well-being data for 2020 used in that report.[344]

However, on 21 April 2022, a study by Butterworth et al was published in Lancet Public Health[345] that uses the HILDA survey data for 2020 to try to isolate the "lockdown effect" by testing the hypothesis that, relative to pre-pandemic levels, the mental health of individuals in the state of Victoria during lockdown (the treatment group) worsened more than that of individuals in the remainder of Australia (the control group). Figure 11.3, taken from the study, shows that both groups experienced a significant decline in this measure of mental health (the "mental health inventory," or "MHI-5").

---

[343] Melbourne Institute, HILDA Statistical Reports. The 15th Annual Statistical Report of the HILDA Survey, https://bit.ly/3OwY7ao.

[344] Melbourne Institute, The 16th Annual Statistical Report of the HILDA Survey, https://bit.ly/3MDvmZy.

[345] Peter Butterworth et al (2022), "Effect of lockdown on mental health in Australia: evidence from a natural experiment analysing a longitudinal probability sample survey," in *The Lancet Public Health*, Volume 7, Issue 5, E427-E436, 1 May 2022, published online on 21 April 2022, DOI: https://doi.org/10.1016/S2468-2667(22)00082-2/fulltext.

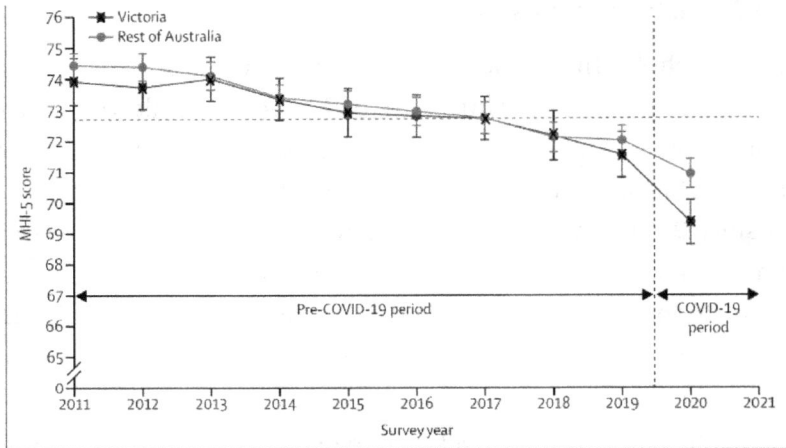

MHI-5 scores range between 0 and 100. Error bars represent 95% CIs. MHI-5=five-item Mental Health Inventory. The horizontal dashed line is the MHI-5 sample mean over the period 2011 to 2020.

Figure 11.3: Mean MHI-5 scores by wave of data collection in Victoria and other Australian states and territories

Mean MHI-5 scores did not differ statistically between the treatment group (72.9 points) and the control group (73.2 points) in the pre-COVID-19 period. In the COVID-19 period, decreased mean scores were seen in both the treatment group (reducing to 69.6 points) and the control group (reducing to 70.8 points). While life satisfaction is different from what is measured by the MHI-5, "the two measures are quite strongly correlated, with the wave specific Pearson correlations ranging from .44 to .49."[346]

The focus of Butterworth et al.'s study was on isolating only the effect of lockdowns, but the overall decline in life satisfaction for all Australians seen above may be due to inescapable elements like some degree of fear plus the range of COVID-excused policies, most notably including lockdowns and border closures but also including measures like masking and social distancing, many of which affected all Australian residents. While awaiting more detailed information from HILDA on life satisfaction during the pandemic, I consider the decline in MHI-5 scores documented in Butterworth et al to be indicative of a moderate fall in life satisfaction in Australia as a whole during 2020.

---

[346] Wooden, M. & Li, N. (2014). "Panel Conditioning and Subjective Well-being," in *Social Indicators Research*, 117 (1), pp. 235-255. https://doi.org/10.1007/s11205-013-0348-1, https://bit.ly/3wN9c01.

11.3.3 *Australian life satisfaction survey: ANUPoll*

ANUPoll[347] is a quarterly survey of Australian public opinion. Illustratively, the 33rd ANUPoll collected information from 3,155 Australians over the period 14-27 April 2020. This survey also has a life satisfaction question. A study by Biddle et al published on 7 May 2020 reported that "Life satisfaction has declined sharply since January 2020 with a drop of 6.90 to 6.50 (out of 10)."[348]

The report of 14 February 2022[349] shows that the average value for life satisfaction in January 2022 was 6.61, far lower than the pre-COVID peak (in October 2019) of 7.05. Figure 11.4 shows the variation in life satisfaction in Australia since October 2019 according to ANUPoll data.

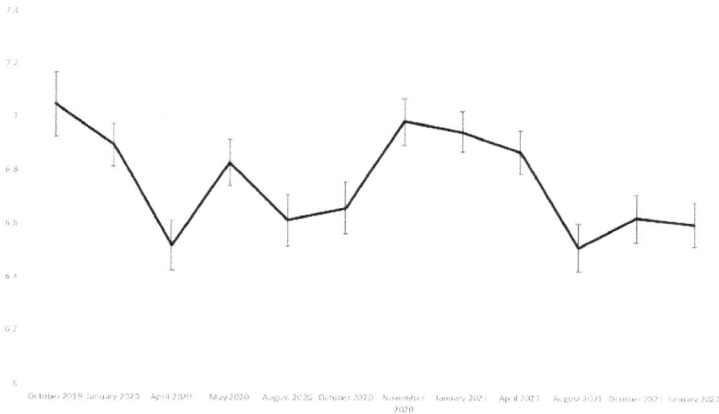

Note: The "whiskers" on the bars indicate the 95 per cent confidence intervals for the estimate.

Source: ANUpoll: October 2019; January, April, May, August, October, and November 2020; January, April, August, and October 2021; and January 2022

Figure 11.4: Life satisfaction in Australia, October 2019 to January 2022

While some data points in Figure 11.4 suggest a loss in life satisfaction of 0.5 points, similar to the result seen early in the UK lockdown period, there is significant variation across months which is likely to

---

[347] Centre for Social Research & Methods, Australian National University. ANU Poll, https://csrm.cass.anu.edu.au/research/surveys/anupoll.

[348] Biddle, Nicholas et al (2020). "Hardship, distress, and resilience: The initial impacts of COVID-19 in Australia," ANUPoll #33 (collected April 2020) – (doi:10.26193/HLMZNW) 7 May 2020, https://bit.ly/3GbMPpt.

[349] Biddle, Nicholas et al (2022). "Tracking wellbeing outcomes during the COVID-19 pandemic (January 2022): Riding the Omicron wave," ANU Centre for Social Research and Methods, https://bit.ly/3wCNehp.

reflect the varying degrees of restrictions imposed during Australia's waves of lockdowns. Based on visual inspection of the ANUPoll data and consistent with the Butterworth et al findings, I consider that a drop in monthly life satisfaction of around 0.3 on average is a reasonable low-range estimate for the impact of the COVID era on Australians' life satisfaction across 2020 and 2021.

We would expect that a country like Sweden – without severe restrictions on movement and without mandatory measures like masking – would have experienced a far smaller drop in life satisfaction. Preliminary data suggest that this might be the case. A 9 June 2021 study on the "Self-Perceived Life Satisfaction during the First Wave of the COVID-19 Pandemic in Sweden"[350] notes that "The Swedish strategy might have contributed to the high proportion of satisfied people."

I therefore attribute the bulk of the documented drop in life satisfaction in Australia, specifically 2/3rds of it, to lockdowns and border closures, viewing 1/3rd of the drop as what would have been experienced in the counterfactual case. I thus estimate that (2/3) x 0.3 = 0.2 is the drop in life satisfaction in Australia that was directly attributable to the lockdowns and border closures implemented in 2020 and 2021.

11.4 The immediate loss of well-being in the currency of WELLBYs

Ignoring any continuing losses in well-being that may be experienced in future by some people subjected to lockdowns, I assume that life satisfaction reduced due to lockdowns only in two years: 2020 and 2021.

By definition, a WELLBY is equal to a one-point increment on a 10-point life satisfaction scale enjoyed for one person for one year. Hence, the total estimated drop in WELLBYs suffered by the 25.7

---

[350] Brogårdh, Christina et al (2021). "Self-Perceived Life Satisfaction during the First Wave of the COVID-19 Pandemic in Sweden: A Cross-Sectional Study," in *Int J Environ Res Public Health*, 2021 Jun; 18(12): 6234, published online 9 June 2021, doi: 10.3390/ijerph18126234, https://www.ncbi.nlm.nih.gov/pmc/articles/PMC8296066/.

million Australian people due to lockdowns equals the estimated decline in life satisfaction of 0.2 (i.e., 20% of a WELLBY) multiplied by 25.7 million, or 5.14 million WELLBYs, in each year.

One year of average healthy life in Australia equates to approximately 6 WELLBYs, so the human cost of this lost life satisfaction is equivalent to the sacrifice of 5.14/6, or 0.8567 million average healthy life-years (QALYs) sacrificed per year of lockdown. This translates to 71,389 QALYs, or **428,334 WELLBYs per month**, for each of years 2020 and 2021.

How many full lives is this worth? A full life is assumed to be 80 years of average healthy life, meaning that the statistical equivalent of [0.8567 million / 80] = 10,707 full lives were lost per year of lockdown through the negative impact of lockdowns on life satisfaction. This translates to 10,707/12 = 892 full lives lost in the average month in 2020 and 2021 due to immediate damage to well-being.

Recognising that an average COVID death represents a sacrifice of 5 remaining healthy life-years (QALYs) (equivalent to 30 WELLBYs), 428,334 WELLBYs per month represents the equivalent of destroying approximately 14,278 (i.e., 428,334/30) lives per month of the type typically lost due to COVID. The fact that these lives were not actually lost (being mental harms) should not make us discount the severity of the impact on Australia of such harms.

11.5 Limitations of this estimate

Life satisfaction measures something that is largely subjective but reflects important aspects of human thriving, such as physical health, mental health, motivation, innovation, bringing up children, social capital and entrepreneurship, among others things. Larger samples and more well-resourced data collection would increase my confidence in the estimates presented above.

The ANUPoll data is robust enough for a ballpark estimate of well-being, but for policy-making purposes one might also like to unpack overall life-satisfaction scores into different types of mental harm. This is left to future research.

12. Mostly future costs: (3) Births, morbidity, mortality, and lifespan

Lockdowns have contributed to a large number of excess (non-COVID) deaths in Australia, as well as to an enormous range of other harms to health and life expectancy beyond the immediate harms to well-being discussed in the previous chapter.

12.1 Mortality, morbidity and lifespan costs in Australia

Some of the costs of lockdowns in relation to heath are outlined below.

Issue	Details	Increased mortality?	Reduced lifespan?
Births	• Children not born because of fewer marriages.[1] • Stillbirths and miscarriages due to fewer medical checkups of pregnant mothers.		
Biological effects	• Epigenetic effects[2] of grief, isolation and stress on pregnant mothers.		✓
Health of children	• Shorter lifespan of children who did not receive timely well-child healthcare during lockdowns (particularly relevant to the disadvantaged segments of Australia's population). • Poorer health due to denial of children's play and the health impacts of forced masking.		✓
Disease identification and treatment	• Fear of catching the virus in hospitals (fed by government messaging) led to delayed presentations for serious medical conditions and delayed routine screenings, leading to delayed detection of disease. • Reduced access to medical care during lockdowns (e.g., restrictions to telehealth rather than in-person consultations, and barriers to GP visits like PCR tests) led to reduced/delayed treatment for many illnesses. • Increased dental disease.[3]	✓	✓

Additional disease burden	• Increased obesity[4] from reduced physical activity, more sitting, troubled sleep, and increased consumption of fast foods and alcohol (fast food outlets and bottle shops were kept open for most of the lockdowns, even as other, healthier food outlets were shut down). Increased obesity is not only a risk factor for death from COVID but also a contributing factor in a wide range of other deaths, e.g., from increased diabetes, in the longer term. In some cases these changes could result in lifelong bad habits, particularly in children.
	
	• Reduced immunity. Lockdowns and border closures reduce immunity in many ways beyond what is covered above – e.g.,:
	
	  ○ border closures reduce the exchange of viruses between people in different regions and overall exposure to and challenge by bioactive agents, thereby reducing immunity over the longer term;[5]
	
	  ○ staying indoors and away from fresh air and sunlight reduces vitamin D levels and hence immunity;
	
	  ○ higher depression and anxiety scores are associated with an enhanced inflammatory state;[6] and
	
	  ○ reduced emotional well-being, social interaction, singing, laughing, wholesome touch, and exercise all reduce immunity
	
	• Some mental harms outlined in the previous chapter may have manifested in an increased medical care burden, e.g., due to increased substance abuse during lockdowns.[7] Psychological and physical trauma from domestic violence, including child abuse, and self-harm could lead to medical conditions.
	
	• Reduced health among the elderly who were prevented from engaging in normal longevity-promoting activities.
		✓	✓

| Increased COVID deaths | • The focus of policy makers on population-wide measures distracted them from the needs of vulnerable cohorts, including those in aged care centres, leading to avoidable COVID deaths. | ✓ | |
| Reduced capacity of health sector | **Reduced funding**
• Reduction in improvements to the average lifespan because the money spent on lockdowns crowded out investments into discovering ways to make life better and longer.
• When GDP and revenue falls, so too does public spending on health-related expenditure items, which translates into more deaths now and in the future.

Reduced staffing
• Health sector disruptions have led to experienced professionals leaving the profession[8] and insufficiently trained junior staff being given senior, independent roles, reducing the quality of diagnosis and treatment. The staff remaining in their roles were likely overworked and took more sick leave, leading to further pressure on the health system, thus further undiagnosed disease and preventable deaths. | ✓ | ✓ |

Notes for Table 1

[1] Marriages plummeted from 113,815 in 2019 to 78,989 in 2020 (Australian Bureau of Statistics. Marriages and Divorces, Australia, 24 November 2021, https://bit.ly/3wB0d20).

[2] Yehuda, Rachel et al (2018). "Intergenerational transmission of trauma effects: putative role of epigenetic mechanisms," in World Psychiatry, 2018 Oct; 17(3): 243–257, https://www.ncbi.nlm.nih.gov/pmc/articles/PMC6127768/.

[3] *ABC News*, "Dentists say teeth grinding has increased during pandemic," 22 November 2021, https://bit.ly/3wPoiT0; *Sydney Morning Herald*, "COVID grind causes 'new pandemic of broken teeth', dentists warn," 11 April 2022, https://bit.ly/3wJp1ov; *The Age*, 'Pushing towards a crisis': Dental waiting lists blow out to record levels, 15 August 2021, https://bit.ly/3lF78C0; Evident Foundation. "COVID-19 restrictions lead to poorer oral health and long-term problems," 14 December 2020, https://bit.ly/3MGWmY6.

[4] *NewsGP*. "One in three Australians have gained weight during the pandemic," 28 January 2021, https://bit.ly/3wLhTb8; Cancer Council WA. "Unintended COVID consequences: Over a third of Aussies gain weight," 22 December 2020, https://bit.ly/3wDsB4N; *Australian Journal of Pharmacy*, "Lockdown Linked to Rise in Gestational Diabetes," 22 September 2021, https://archive.ph/vTada.

⁵ E.g., as reported in *The Guardian*, "New Zealand children falling ill in high numbers due to Covid 'immunity debt'," 8 July 2021, https://bit.ly/3NtWxGe.

⁶ Shafiee, Mojtaba et al (2017). "Depression and anxiety symptoms are associated with white blood cell count and red cell distribution width: A sex-stratified analysis in a population-based study," in Psychoneuroendocrinology, October 2017, 84:101-108. doi: 10.1016/j.psyneuen.2017.06.021.

⁷ "CSIRO study reveals COVID-19's impact on weight and emotional wellbeing," 16 June 2020, https://bit.ly/3MwFjYB.

⁸ *GoodRxHealth* reported on "The Impact of COVID-19 on Healthcare Careers," 28 April 2022, https://archive.ph/l0kBD; the *Sydney Morning Herald* reported similarly: "Pandemic triggers 'mass exodus' of critical care nurses," 17 November 2021, https://bit.ly/3wFbL5H.

Detection of cancers has been a key concern given the impotance of early detection in achieving successful treatment for cancer. According to oncologist Karol Sikoa, former director of the WHO's cancer program, "catching cancer at the earlier stages usually means roughly an 80% or more survival rate. At later stages, that drops to around 20%."[351] Remote consultation by GPs does not work as well as in-person visits for cancer screening and other types of diagnostic health checks:

> An official assessment by the Department of Health and Social Care (DHSC) and the Office for National Statistics (ONS) revealed the "unintended consequences" of resorting to remote consultations. More than 175,000 diagnoses of key conditions are estimated to have been missed in 2020, the document states.[352]

In addition to the health harms outlined above, in some countries there were additional homicides during lockdowns: "According to Dame Vera Baird, victims' commissioner in the U.K., domestic-abuse murders of women increased significantly, possibly doubled, during lockdown."[353] In addition, more violence against babies was observed. The BBC reported on 7 November 2020 that:

> There was an alarming 20% rise in babies being killed or

---

[351] Tweet dated 27 September 2021 by Karol Sikora, https://archive.ph/GHjyM.

[352] *The Telegraph*. "GPs demand more cash to see patients face-to-face," 17 September 2021, https://bit.ly/3NwMNeo.

[353] Grierson, Jamie (2020). "Domestic abuse killings 'more than double' amid Covid-19 lockdown," in *The Guardian*, 14 April 2020, https://bit.ly/3PyHAo2.

harmed during the first lockdown, Ofsted's chief inspector Amanda Spielman has revealed. Sixty-four babies were deliberately harmed in England – eight of whom died. Some 40% of the 300 incidents reported involved infants, up a fifth on 2019. Ms Spielman believes a "toxic mix" of isolation, poverty and mental illness caused the March to October spike. Health staff and social workers were hampered by Covid restrictions. And many regular visits could not take place, while others were carried out remotely, using the telephone or video links.[354]

However, data on homicides in Australia for 2020 are now available, and there were fewer total homicides in Australia under lockdowns, an effect already captured on the "benefit" side in this report.

12.2 Health harms in developing nations

The developing world suffered significant damage from COVID lockdowns. To the extent that policymakers in developing countries followed the lead of developed countries, Australia also bears some responsibility for the vast lockdown harms experienced in developing countries.

According to the WHO, at least 100,000 additional people died because of lockdowns only from tuberculosis in 2020, with additional deaths likely to be worse in 2021 and 2022 since thousands have not been properly diagnosed as resources were diverted from standard diseases to COVID. The number of people newly diagnosed with TB and reported to national governments fell from 7.1 million in 2019 to 5.8 million in 2020.[355]

Gerd Muller, German Minister of Economic Cooperation and Development, said on 25 September 2020[356] that lockdowns have resulted in "one of the biggest" hunger and poverty crises in history. He

---

[354] *BBC News*, "'Toxic lockdown' sees huge rise in babies harmed or killed," 6 November 2020, https://bit.ly/39MMbT1.

[355] World Health Organization. Global Tuberculosis Report 2021, 14 October 2021, https://archive.ph/ilVvK.

[356] Durden, Tyler (2020). "German Minister Admits Lockdown Will Kill More Than COVID-19 Does," in *Zerohedge*, 26 September 2020, https://archive.ph/XAgse.

estimated that "an additional 400,000 deaths from malaria and HIV" would occur in 2020 "on the African continent alone." Further, "half a million more will die from tuberculosis." These deaths are largely attributable to the breakdown in supply of food and medication and a lack of funding from Western aid programs.

Some reports suggest disruptions in birth safety in developing countries. UNICEF has warned that disruptions arising from lockdowns could result in potentially devastating increases in maternal and child deaths.[357] A *Lancet* study reported a 50% increase in stillbirths during lockdowns in developing countries because of insufficient medical care.[358]

Professor Ramesh Thakur of the Australian National University wrote on 24 October 2020:

> Of course, the biggest tragedy will be across the developing world over the next decade, with over 100 million more people pushed into extreme poverty, tens of millions of additional dead from increased infant and maternal mortality, hunger and starvation with more poverty and disrupted crop production and food distribution networks, sharp cutbacks in immunisation and schooling, and destruction of the informal sectors of the economy in which daily wage earners earn a pitiful living. Most countries will also need to prepare for potential spikes in mental health problems and suicides from the fear generated by exaggerated alarmism as well as the loneliness, isolation, financial ruin and despair caused by the lockdowns.[359]

The Harvard School of Public Health reported on 23 June 2021 that health care providers in Africa reported that more than half (56%) of essential health care services – including child and maternal

[357] UNICEF (2020). "As COVID-19 devastates already fragile health systems, over 6,000 additional children under five could die a day, without urgent action," Press Release, 12 May 2020, https://archive.ph/dyQnF.
[358] Watson, Clare (2020). "Stillbirth rate rises dramatically during pandemic," in *Nature*, 15 September 2020, https://www.nature.com/articles/d41586-020-02618-5.
[359] Thakur, Ramesh (2020). "Hippocrates cancelled," in *Spectator Australia*, 24 October 2020, https://bit.ly/3wED13W.

nutrition and health services, HIV treatment, and surgeries – were disrupted due to COVID-19 restrictions.[360]

In addition, there have been many reports of a significant drop-off in childhood vaccinations in developing countries.[361] It was reported on 23 September 2021 that:

> Mission Indradhanush, one of India's immunization programs responsible for administering vaccinations to 26 million children 29 million pregnant women [sic] every year, saw its community-based delivery activities levelled. A 40% increase in child mortality due to vaccine-preventable illness is expected if its course is not righted (Shet et al., 2021).[362]

In an article in the *New York Times* on 28 October 2021,[363] Benjamin Mueller noted that "The pandemic dealt a serious setback to global efforts to immunize children against diseases like measles and polio. The proportion of eligible children who received a polio vaccine fell to 83 percent in 2020 from 86 percent the year before, as did coverage with the third dose of the diphtheria-tetanus-pertussis vaccine, known as DTP3. Coverage with the measles vaccine also dipped slightly, to 84 percent last year from 86 percent in 2019. Those setbacks, while seemingly small, meant that millions more children missed out on routine immunizations during the pandemic, putting them and their communities at risk."

Below is a lightly edited table taken from a 2021 paper by Ari Joffe summarising the harms of lockdowns in the developing world.[364] While this table is focused on harms in developing nations, harms similar to some of these have also occurred in Australia, particularly among disadvantaged people.

[360] *EurekaAlert.* "COVID-19 disruptions in sub-Saharan Africa will have substantial health consequences," 23 June 2021, https://www.eurekalert.org/news-releases/913486
[361] World Health Organization. "WHO and UNICEF warn of a decline in vaccinations during COVID-19," 15 July 2020, https://archive.ph/x2bM6.
[362] Collateral Global. "Global Catastrophe," 23 September 2021, https://archive.ph/8nvqI.
[363] *New York Times* (2021). "Childhood vaccinations have lagged across the world because of the pandemic," 28 October 2021, https://bit.ly/3wJdZQb.
[364] https://www.frontiersin.org/articles/10.3389/fpubh.2021.625778/full, Joffe, A. (2021). "COVID-19: Rethinking the Lockdown Groupthink," in *Frontiers in Public Health*, 9, 98. fpubh.2021.625778.

Sustainable Development Goal	Effect of COVID-19 Response
Childhood Vaccination	Programs stalled in 70 countries [Measles, Diphtheria, Cholera, Polio]
Education	- School Closures: 90% of students (1.57 billion) kept out of school - Early primary grades are most vulnerable, with effects into adulthood: effects on outcomes of intelligence, teen pregnancy, illicit drug use, graduation rates, employment rates and earnings, arrest rates, hypertension, diabetes mellites, depression - Not just education affected: school closures have effects on food security, loss of a place of safety, less physical activity, lost social interaction, lost support services for developmental difficulties, economic effects on families
Sexual and reproductive health services	Lack of access: estimated ~ 2.7 million unsafe abortions For every 3 months of lockdown, estimated 2 million more lack access to contraception, and over 6 months, 7 million more additional unintended pregnancies
Food security	Hunger Pandemic: undernourished estimate to increase 83 to 132 million (>225,000/day) – from disrupted food chains supplies (labor mobility, food transport, planting seasons] and access to food [from job losses and incomes, price increases]
End Poverty	Extreme Poverty (Living on <$1.90 per day): Estimated to increase >70 million – Lost "ladders of opportunity" and social determinants of health
Reduce Maternal and Under-5 mortality	Estimated increase of 1.16 million children (USM) and 56,700 maternal deaths, if essential Reproductive Maternal Newborn and Child Health services are disrupted (coverage reduction 39-52%) for 6 months in 188 Low- and Middle-Income Countries. Mostly (~60%) due to affected childhood interventions (wasting, antibiotics, ORS115 for diarrhea); and childbirth interventions (uterotonics, antibiotics, anticonvulsants, clean birth)
Infectious Disease Mortality	Tuberculosis: in moderate/severe scenario, projected excess deaths 342,000-1.36 Million over 5 years Malaria: in moderate/severe scenario, projected excess deaths 203,000 to 415,000 over 1 year HIV: In moderate scenario, projected deaths 296,000 (range 229,000-420,000) in Sub-Saharan Africa over 1 year (an increase of 63%). Also, would increase mother-to-child transmission by 1.5 times

In my book, *The Great Covid Panic*, my co-authors and I discuss Ari Joffe's table. I reproduce our discussion below.

This table only counts physical health effects due to disruptions that took place in the Illusion of Control phase. It considers both short-run and long-run effects. Each of the claimed effects is based on a published study about that effect.

First on the list is the disruption to vaccination programs for measles, diphtheria, cholera, and polio, which were either cancelled or reduced in scope in some 70 countries. That disruption was caused by travel restrictions. Western experts could not travel, and within many poor countries travel and general activity were also halted in the early days of the Illusion of Control phase. This depressive effect on vaccination programs for the poor is expected to lead to large loss of life in the coming years. The poor countries paying this cost are most countries in Africa, the poorer nations in Asia, such as India, Indonesia and Myanmar, and the poorer countries in Latin America.

The second listed effect in the table relates to schooling. An estimated 90% of the world's children have had their schooling disrupted, often for months, which reduces their lifetime opportunities and social development through numerous direct and indirect pathways. The UN children's organisation, UNICEF, has released several reports on just how bad the consequences of this will be in the coming decades.

The third element in Joffe's table refers to reports of economic and social primitivisation in poor countries. Primitivisation, also seen after the collapse of the Soviet Union in the early 1990s, is just what it sounds like: a regression away from specialisation, trade and economic advancement through markets to more isolated and 'primitive' choices, including attempted economic self-sufficiency and higher fertility. Due to diminished labour market prospects, curtailed educational activities and decreased access to reproductive health services, populations in the Illusion of Control phase began reverting to having more children precisely in those countries where there is already huge pressure on resources.

The fourth and fifth elements listed in the table reflect the biggest disaster of this period, namely the increase in extreme poverty and expected famines in poor countries. Over the 20 years leading up to 2020, gradual improvements in economic conditions around the world had significantly eased poverty and famines. Now, international organisations are signalling rapid deterioration in both. The Food and Agriculture Organisation (FAO) now expects the world to have approximately an additional 100 million extremely poor people facing starvation as a result of Covid policies. That will translate into civil wars, waves of refugees and huge loss of life.

The last two items in Joffe's table relate to the effect of lower perinatal and infant care and impoverishment. Millions of preventable deaths are now expected due to infections and weakness in new mothers and young infants, and neglect of other health problems like malaria and tuberculosis that affect people in all walks of life. The whole of the poor world has suffered fewer than one million deaths from Covid. The price to be paid in human losses in these countries through hunger and health neglect caused by lockdowns and other restrictions is much, much larger. All in the name of stopping Covid.

Ari Joffe's table highlights many uncomfortable truths. One is that the single-minded attention to the development of vaccines against Covid – over 200 and counting – could have been spent instead on research and direct efforts on the ground directed at preventing or treating much more dangerous diseases, such as tuberculosis, cholera or malaria.

Many other harms of lockdowns were seen in developing countries. One example is child trafficking. Professor Ramesh Thakur of the Australian National University wrote on 24 October 2020:

> I ask the question 'triggered' by a report in the Indian Express (12 October). There's been a sharp surge in child trafficking in India following lockdowns. Westerners have forgotten what 'hand to mouth' existence means, when the

sole breadwinner must earn daily wages to buy food for the family, including elderly parents. With lockdown for months without end, children are inevitably at risk of being trafficked into labour bondage, street begging or sexual slavery.

12.3 Evidence of health harms of lockdowns in Australia and elsewhere in the developed world

I now provide a snapshot of the empirical evidence of the kinds of harms outlined above that were witnessed in the developed world.

12.3.1 Delayed presentations and increased backlog

During the COVID pandemic, health care for problems other than COVID was often delayed or fully crowded out. It was reported on 14 April 2020 by *NewsGP*, the news hub of the Royal Australian College of General Practitioners, that presentations at hospitals and general practices across Australia had dropped by around 50% across the board. Moreover, there were "worrying declines of up to 50% in new cancer patients and 30% in cardiac emergencies, according to Victorian experts."[365]

According to a 26 September 2020 news report:

> Cardiac-arrest survival rates halved in Victoria during the first wave of the coronavirus pandemic. The spike in deaths has been linked to a sharp decline in bystanders performing CPR on the street and a lack of access to the state's more than 6500 public defibrillators which are stored in shuttered schools, offices, sporting clubs and shopping centres. "We have seen fluctuations of 1, 2 or 3 per cent, but we are talking about a fluctuation of around 50 per cent". If this trend continues, researchers estimate an extra 186 preventable cardiac arrest deaths will occur this year.[366]

It was reported on 11 September 2020 in *ABC News*[367] that in Victoria:

---

[365] *NewsGP*. "Drastic drop in cancer and heart attack patients linked to COVID-19," 14 April 2020, https://bit.ly/3wCIHvz.

[366] *Sydney Morning Herald*. "'I couldn't let a mate die': Study shows hidden spike in cardiac deaths," 26 September 2020, https://bit.ly/38F8078.

[367] *ABC News*. "Cancer screening, heart attack and stroke presentations down in Victoria during coronavirus pandemic," 11 September 2020, https://bit.ly/3MHr7vT.

Hospitals are reporting a 'concerning' decline in the number of Victorians seeking treatment for heart attacks and strokes, as well as essential cancer screening, during the state's coronavirus second wave. Health Minister Jenny Mikakos said the number of people presenting to emergency departments with strokes was down 24 per cent on the same time last year. For heart attacks, the number of ED presentations was down 18 per cent. "This does suggest that people are putting off seeking urgent and important medical care that could make that critical difference to their life," Ms Mikakos said.

The report noted that: "Victoria has seen a 30 per cent drop in reports for the five most common cancers."

Cancer screenings and presentations of heart disease and stroke all declined in Victoria in the middle months of 2020.[368] There were early reports in Australia of additional cancer deaths.[369]

While detailed data on Australians' GP visits is not readily available, data from the USA provides a guide.[370] It shows that there was a significant cumulative decline in visits to medical specialists, ranging from 27% for pediatrics to 8% for rheumatology. There was a 20% reduction in visits to cardiologists and a 13% reduction in visits to oncologists.

By the end of June 2020, an estimated 41% of US adults had delayed or avoided medical care.[371] A significant drop-off was observed in diabetes patients picking up their prescribed medicines.[372]

---

[368] *ABC News.* "Cancer screening, heart attack and stroke presentations down in Victoria during coronavirus pandemic," 11 September 2020, https://bit.ly/3MHr7vT.

[369] Scholefield, Antony (2020). "Pandemic shutdown 'means thousands more bowel cancer deaths," in *AusDoc,* 21 September 2020. https://bit.ly/39QrA0s.

[370] Mehrotra, Ateev, et al (2021). "The Impact of COVID-19 on Outpatient Visits in 2020: Visits Remained Stable, Despite a Late Surge in Cases," Commonwealth Fund, 22 February 2021, https://bit.ly/3NrjppG

[371] Czeisler, M.É. et al, "Delay or Avoidance of Medical Care Because of COVID-19–Related Concerns – United States, June 2020," in *MMWR Morb Mortal Wkly Rep* 2020;69:1250–1257. https://bit.ly/3wzkJ4i.

[372] Yunusa, Ismaeel (2021). "Fewer diabetes patients are picking up their insulin prescriptions – another way the pandemic has delayed health care for many," in *The Conversation,* 12 November 2021, https://bit.ly/38HwIne.

On 14 October 2020, Dr Scott Atlas estimated that 46% of cancers had not been diagnosed due to lockdowns, 50% of chemotherapy appointments had been missed, 50% of immunisations had been missed and 25% of young people had considered suicide.[373]

A Canadian newspaper reported as follows on 24 October 2020, leading with a quote from a cancer surgeon: "'Anecdotally, we are seeing more advanced cancers as patients finally present to their surgical specialist,' he said, noting that usually means patients will require a bigger operation and longer hospital stay and are more likely to need radiation and chemotherapy and other multidisciplinary care. "So the impact to the entire system is significant."[374]

Professor Ramesh Thakur of the Australian National University wrote as follows on 24 October 2020:

> 'Hundreds of thousands of cancer screenings were deferred after worries about Covid-19 shut down much of the US health-care system this spring', the *Wall Street Journal* reported on 15 October. 'There's really almost no way that doesn't turn into increased mortality'.[375]

The Canadian newspaper article quoted above went on to report the following on 24 October 2020:[376]

> Between March 15 and May 31, screenings for all three cancers plunged compared to the same period in 2019. According to data shared by Ontario Health, there was a 97 per cent decrease in screening mammograms (4,065 from 158,967), an 88 per cent decrease in Pap tests (26,269 from 219,079) and a 73 per cent decrease in fecal tests (38,000 from 141,251) in provincial programs.

On 29 October 2020 another report entitled "Cancer crisis: The

---

[373] Tweet dated 14 October 2020 by Justin Hart, https://archive.ph/eWjKN.

[374] *Toronto Star* (2020). "Ontario shut down non-urgent health services in the spring. Now hospitals are seeing many more patients with advanced cancers," 24 October 2020, https://bit.ly/3Nun7Pj.

[375] Thakur, Ramesh (2020). "Hippocrates cancelled," in *Spectator Australia*, 24 October 2020, https://bit.ly/3wED13W.

[376] *Toronto Star* (2020). "Ontario shut down non-urgent health services in the spring. Now hospitals are seeing many more patients with advanced cancers," 24 October 2020, https://bit.ly/3Nun7Pj.

hidden victims of COVID – 50,000 people missing a diagnosis" noted that:

> "As the pandemic escalated, we know there was a significant drop in people visiting their GP with symptoms and being referred for cancer tests. This has meant a 'colossal' 50,000 people in the UK are now missing a cancer diagnosis because of the disruptions caused by COVID-19 – a number that could double by this time next year."[377]

It was reported on 29 October 2020 that Richard Sullivan, Professor of cancer and global health at King's College London and director of its Institute for Cancer Policy, opined that '[t]he number of deaths due to the disruption of cancer services is likely to outweigh the number of deaths from the coronavirus itself. The cessation and delay of cancer care will cause considerable avoidable suffering. Cancer screening services have stopped, which means we will miss our chance to catch many cancers when they are treatable and curable, such as cervical, bowel and breast. When we do restart normal service delivery after the lockdown is lifted, the backlog of cases will be a huge challenge to the healthcare system."[378]

On 30 March 2021 a report on a survey by the American Society for Radiation Oncology said that the "COVID-19 pandemic has led to more advanced-stage cancer diagnoses."[379]

A 29 April 2021 study in *JAMA Oncology* reported "an estimated screening deficit of 9.4 million associated with the COVID-19 pandemic for the US population."[380]

A study published on 26 May 2021 reported that in the US, "over-

---

[377] *Express.* "Cancer crisis: The hidden victims of COVID – 50,000 people missing a diagnosis," 29 October 2020, https://bit.ly/3MyOzLP.

[378] Durden, Tyler (2020). "This Isn't Human!" – The 'Unseen' Perils Of COVID From "A Faceless Number In Melbourne," in ZeroHedge, 29 October 2020, https://bit.ly/3wMzXl8.

[379] ASTRO. "COVID-19 pandemic has led to more advanced-stage cancer diagnoses, physician survey finds," 30 March 2021, https://bit.ly/3ySusnP.

[380] Chen, Robert et al (2021). "Association of Cancer Screening Deficit in the United States With the COVID-19 Pandemic," in *JAMA Oncol.* 2021;7(6):878-884. doi:10.1001/jama-oncol.2021.0884, https://jamanetwork.com/journals/jamaoncology/fullarticle/2778916.

dose-associated cardiac arrests rose about 40% nationally in 2020, with the largest increases among racial/ethnic minorities, in areas of socioeconomic disadvantage."[381]

A 3 June 2021 report notes: "There was a 40% decline in the number of patients admitted with heart attacks (acute coronary syndromes) in 2020" in the UK.[382]

On 28 June 2021 a report noted the findings of a study that appeared in *The Journal of the National Cancer Institute*, which found a 10.2% decline in real-time electronic pathology reports from population-based cancer registries in 2020 compared with 2019. This study observation period, through December 2020, was one of the longest to date that has evaluated the effects of the COVID-19 pandemic on cancer-related trends.[383]

On 14 July 2021 a report on a study noted that "By 2030, the models project 950 additional breast cancer deaths related to reduced screening; 1,314 associated with delayed diagnosis of symptomatic cases, and 151 due to reduced chemotherapy use in women with early stage breast cancer. This corresponds to a 0.52% increase in breast cancer deaths between 2020 and 2030."[384]

On 26 November 2021 a news report noted:

> Research by Macmillan Cancer Support shows a "staggering" backlog of cases that have yet to be diagnosed, with concern that services are buckling even before the unmet need is addressed. It estimated that more than 47,000 people have "missed" a diagnosis in the UK since the first lockdown. It ... estimated that the NHS in England would need to work at 110 per cent capacity for 13 months in a row to

---

[381] Friedman, Joseph et al (2021). "Racial/Ethnic, Social, and Geographic Trends in Overdose-Associated Cardiac Arrests Observed by US Emergency Medical Services During the COVID-19 Pandemic," in *JAMA Psychiatry*. 2021;78(8):886–895. doi:10.1001/jamapsychiatry.2021.0967, https://jamanetwork.com/journals/jamapsychiatry/fullarticle/2780427.

[382] University of Exeter, 3 June 2021, https://archive.ph/TSEVa.

[383] EurekAlert! "Study finds adverse effects of COVID-19 pandemic on cancer detection and surgical treatments," 28 June 2021, https://www.eurekalert.org/news-releases/862525.

[384] EurekAlert! "COVID precautions may result in more breast cancer deaths," 14 July 2021, https://www.eurekalert.org/news-releases/745072.

catch up with the number of people who should have started cancer treatment since March 2020.[385]

It was reported by the BBC on 24 September 2021 that:

> it could take more than a decade to clear the cancer-treatment backlog in England, a report suggests. Research by the Institute for Public Policy Research estimated 19,500 people who should have been diagnosed had not been, because of missed referrals. If hospitals could achieve a 5% increase in the number of treatments over pre-pandemic levels, it would take until 2033 to clear the backlog. But if 15% more could be completed, backlogs could be cleared by next year."[386]

12.3.2 *Active decisions to reduce treatment of non-COVID issues*

Governments shut down some essential treatments to prioritise COVID in 2020 and 2021, even though hospitals appeared to have sufficient capacity.[387] For example, the UK Health Secretary Matt Hancock said on 6 October 2020 that cancer treatment would have to wait until the coronavirus was 'under control.'[388] A news article of 10 September 2021[389] reported that Professor David Baldwin, chair of the Lung Cancer Clinical Expert Group, said that guidance from the Prime Minister's office discouraged people with a hallmark symptom of lung cancer from seeking medical help. "It kept

---

[385] *The Telegraph*. "'Staggering' backlog of missed cancer diagnoses could hit 50,000," 26 November 2021, https://archive.ph/Vx8CP.

[386] *BBC News*. "Covid: Cancer backlog could take a decade to clear," 24 September 2021, https://bit.ly/388rAbq.

[387] On 10 December 2020, when it was going through its second peak of COVID cases, "Sweden still [had] 148 unoccupied beds in intensive care wards nationwide, corresponding to 22% free capacity" (Reuters, "Sweden sets new daily COVID case record, says ICU beds not full," 11 December 2020, https://archive.ph/hRcVU). In Australia, COVID cases never reached significant levels until late 2021. Some evidence about ICU capacity can be gleaned from an ABC report of 2 September 2021 which showed that Victoria had a potential capacity of 1200 ICU beds but from August to October 2021, the peak ICU usage for COVID patients was 157 (ABC, "How many COVID cases can Victoria handle before its hospitals' ICU capacity is overrun?," https://archive.ph/W3T7m.

[388] Thakur, Ramesh (2020). "Hippocrates cancelled," in *Spectator Australia*, 24 October 2020, https://bit.ly/3wED13W.

[389] *Daily Mail*. "Telling patients with coughs to stay away from the NHS during the Covid pandemic put lung cancer care back up to 25 YEARS, experts tell MPs," 9 November 2021, https://bit.ly/3NyoxIv.

lung cancer patients at home more often so we saw a 69 per cent reduction in referrals." The report noted that lung cancer has a five-year survival rate of 57 percent if caught early, but only 3 percent if found late.

There is evidence that in Australia some medical tests were temporarily suspended to focus on COVID. For example, the Faecal Multiplex PCR, which can detect 13 enteric pathogens responsible for both viral and protozoal gastroenteritis, was not provided to a patient, with COVID used as the excuse.[390]

12.3.3 Increased disorders among the young

A 12 November 2021 report noted that in the UK, "Covid killed just six healthy children during the pandemic, while lockdowns have fuelled a timebomb of health disorders among the young."[391] Developed nations, like Canada, have seen advanced cancers in children due to delayed or missed screenings during lockdowns:[392] "As a pediatric doctor, Singh says that it has been heartbreaking to see some of the children whose cancers have progressed much further than the pre-pandemic norm."

On 16 November 2021 a report in *The Telegraph* showed that childhood obesity increased significantly during lockdowns. The following data[393] are from the UK.

> Among reception-aged children – those aged four and five – the rates of obesity rose from 9.9 per cent in 2019/20 to 14.4 per cent in 2020/21.
>
> For those aged 10 and 11, who are in their last year of primary school, obesity prevalence increased from 21 per cent to 25.5 per cent.

---

[390] The redacted image of an email received by a person from a Victorian pathology lab is shown on page 121 of a complaint by Sanjeev Sabhlok to the International Criminal Court (https://bit.ly/3yT7HAm).

[391] *The Telegraph* (2021). "Six healthy children died of Covid in a year, but lockdowns fuel youth health timebomb," 12 November 2021, https://bit.ly/3MJ5Q5c.

[392] *CBC*. "Late diagnosis of tumours in children collateral damage of COVID-19, doctors say," 21 November 2021, https://archive.ph/bZArx.

[393] *The Telegraph* (2021). "Lockdowns fuel 'alarming' rise in child obesity," 16 November 2021, https://archive.ph/OfliZ.

It means that overall, 27.7 per cent of pupils were overweight or obese by the age of five, compared with 23 per cent the year before.

As a result of the dysfunction of the health system in the UK, a news report on 16 November 2021 in *The Telegraph* noted: "Nearly 10,000 more people than usual have died in the past four months from non-Covid reasons, as experts called for an urgent government inquiry into whether the deaths were preventable."[394] A similar tragedy did not happen in Sweden, where there were no excess deaths in 2021 and no excessive pressure on the health system.

12.3.4 *Domestic border closures led to the deaths of babies*

On 18 October 2020 it was reported that four newborns in Adelaide had died after being denied lifesaving heart surgery that required interstate transfers disallowed because of travel restrictions.[395] This was confirmed in *The Australian* newspaper on 21 October 2020: "Victoria's stage-four lockdown prevented four sick newborn babies – who subsequently died – from being flown from Adelaide to Melbourne to receive lifesaving cardiac surgery."[396]

12.3.5 *Increases in the prevalence and impact of chronic illnesses*

On 16 November 2021, the BBC reported: "When the pandemic hit, about a quarter of adults in the UK were living with chronic illnesses. With support and care disrupted and Covid making people more isolated and less active, their health has suffered. According to those working in the NHS, they are now turning up to hospital in ever greater numbers."[397] Another BBC news report on the same date noted, "At the end of September, 64,962 people in England waited

---

[394] *The Telegraph* (2021). "Alarm grows as mortuaries fill with thousands of extra non-Covid deaths," 16 November 2021, https://archive.ph/jI26H.

[395] Tweet dated 21 October 2020 by Simon Dolan, https://bit.ly/3LDoCta.

[396] Penberthy, David (2020). "Coronavirus: Why were these four newborns left to die?" in *The Australian*, 21 October 2020, https://bit.ly/3GbPGi5.

[397] *BBC News*. "Why the NHS is struggling like never before," 16 November 2021, https://archive.ph/CC8zZ

more than six weeks for heart ultrasounds (known as echocardiograms), compared to 3,238 people who waited this long at the end of February 2020."[398]

Many normal health and welfare services were disrupted because resources were re-allocated to COVID. For example, in the UK, children's commissioner Koulla Yiasouma noted that:

> Health visitors were redeployed to provide Covid-19 related care and services resulting in a reduction in the number of health assessments and home visits. Reductions in health visiting appointments, in addition to restrictions in access to other early years services, removed an important support system for parents, particularly first-time mothers and those from disadvantaged backgrounds.[399]

Amanda Brumwell reported on Collateral Global that:

> restrictions in the provision of care further limited the number of people able to secure routine services even if they calculated the relative risk appropriately. Such restrictions, which do not even include restrictions in individual mobility that likely complicated health seeking behaviors, amounted to the weeks- or months-long closure of community clinics and stoppage of outpatient services at larger health facilities across the globe. In some government clinics where our organization works, we were informed that no admittance was allowed at all unless it was for a COVID-19 positive person, for extended periods of time. The impact was horrifying for those suffering with acute effects of TB, diabetes, and accidents, and for childhood vaccination the damage will be similar – both short- and long-term damage are sure to follow from children unprotected from infections that drive mortality among them in poorer settings.[400]

---

[398] *BBC News*. "Record numbers waiting over six weeks for vital heart scans," 16 November 2021, https://archive.ph/frH5m.

[399] *BBC News*. "Covid-19: Pandemic had severe impact on young people, says report," 26 August 2021, https://archive.ph/PAhAi

[400] Collateral Global. "Global Catastrophe," 23 September 2021, https://archive.ph/8nvqI.

12.3.6 *Reduced physical activity and increased obesity*

A 17 September 2021 report[401] shows the change in body mass index (BMI) in different American cohorts. Younger children suffered the most from lack of exercise during lockdowns. To the extent that these effects are permanent, the longevity of these children will be reduced.

A 2021 survey showed that "35% of Australians have gained weight … Ipsos Australia Director, David Elliott said that it 'isn't surprising' that one third of Australians surveyed reported weight gain during the pandemic."[402] Another study has shown that "Australians gained average of three kilograms over pandemic."[403] "A further survey by the CSIRO found Australian adults reported having gained three to five kilograms during the first lockdown."[404]

Global data point in a similar direction: "in a study by Dragun et al., 27.3% of respondents increased their intake of sweets and snacks during lockdown. In a Canadian study by Carroll et al more than half of the respondents felt that their diet had changed since COVID-19: the most common changes included eating more food."[405]

Gym closures likely implied changes to regular exercise routines:

> Midday, 23 March 2020 will forever be etched in the memory of fitness facilities, exercise professionals and fitness industry staff as a day that more than 6,400 fitness businesses

---

[401] Lange, Samantha J. et al (2021). "Longitudinal Trends in Body Mass Index Before and During the COVID-19 Pandemic Among Persons Aged 2–19 Years – United States, 2018–2020," in *Morbidity and Mortality Weekly Report*, Centres for Disease Control and Prevention, 17 September 2021, https://bit.ly/3tekqdh.

[402] *NewsGP*. "One in three Australians have gained weight during the pandemic," 28 January 2021, https://bit.ly/3wLhTb8.

[403] SiSU Health. "Australians gained average of three kilograms over pandemic, new data shows," 29 June 2021, https://archive.ph/vXmvf.

[404] Macquarie University (The Lighthouse). "How to kick those COVID kilos for good," 29 March 2021, https://archive.ph/TtBp7.

[405] Białek-Dratwa, Agnieszka et al (2022). "Health Behaviors and Associated Feelings of Remote Workers During the COVID-19 Pandemic – Silesia (Poland)" in *Front. Public Health*, 27 January 2022, https://www.frontiersin.org/articles/10.3389/fpubh.2022.774509/full.

closed indefinitely, put more than 35,000 people immediately out of work and removed the option of gym-based exercise from 4 million Australians.[406]

However, with the end of lockdowns, this has been improving:

Fortunately, it is being reported that by January 2022 in a particular example, "We've had more than half our clients return and we've signed up more new members in the past two-and-a-half months than we did in whole 2020 [sic] calendar year." (*ibid*)

Further examples of harms in these areas from lockdowns are provided at the web addresses below.

a) Reduced exercise and fitness:

- https://www.eurekalert.org/pub_releases/2021-05/aru-lma051921.php
- https://www.eurekalert.org/pub_releases/2021-06/fda-loe063021.php
- https://www.eurekalert.org/pub_releases/2021-05/guf-pal052721.php

b) Obesity and eating:

- https://www.eurekalert.org/pub_releases/2021-05/uodc-sda052721.php

12.3.7 *Excess non-COVID deaths*

An estimate was made in late 2020, based on official statistics, that lockdowns would lead to around 100,000 additional (non-COVID) deaths in the US.[407] *The Lancet* published a paper[408] on 10 August 2020 showing an increase in excess deaths from non-COVID causes:

---

[406] AUSactive. "Fitness industry continues to strengthen 12 months since COVID-19 shutdowns," 22 March 2021, https://archive.ph/j9AQa.

[407] Tweet dated 23 October by Ethical Skeptic, https://archive.ph/dQHH3.

[408] https://www.thelancet.com/journals/lanpub/article/PIIS2468-2667(20)30180-8/fulltext, Pell, Robert et al (2020). "Coronial autopsies identify the indirect effects of COVID-19," in *The Lancet Public Health*, 10 August 2020.

Indirect increases in morbidity and mortality resulting from movement restrictions imposed during the COVID-19 pandemic have been identified as a public health concern. Deaths registered in England and Wales exceeded the 5-year average by almost 50 000 during the first 2 months of lockdown.

A 25 August 2020 UK report stated that the Health Data Research Hub for Cancer had "used health data to predict that there could potentially be an additional 18,000 additional deaths in people with cancer, as a result of the pandemic."[409]

On 2 September 2020, *The Telegraph* reported that "Patients dying at home from causes other than Covid-19 are fuelling excess deaths across the UK. The data from the Office for National Statistics shows more than 6,700 extra deaths in homes across the UK in the past two months."[410]

Professor Ramesh Thakur of the Australian National University wrote on 24 October 2020:

> The US Centres for Disease Control estimates 93,814 non-Covid excess American deaths. In the UK, 'up to 150,000' could suffer non-Covid-19 premature deaths, the Financial Times reported.[411]

In May 2022, the World Health Organization published a report estimating 14.9 million excess deaths globally with only 5.42 million of them being reported as COVID deaths. It noted that this figure of 14.9 million "also includes deaths indirectly associated with COVID-19, due to other causes and diseases, resulting from the wider impact of the pandemic on health systems and society."[412] The only country without lockdowns, Sweden, had fewer excess deaths

[409] Health Data Research UK (2020). "The Big C isn't COVID-19 - it's cancer," 25 August 2020, https://bit.ly/3wL2FmI.

[410] Donnelly, Laura (2020). "Non-virus deaths at home behind surge in excess fatalities, figures show," in *The Telegraph*, 2 September 2020. https://bit.ly/39LnDtz.

[411] Thakur, Ramesh (2020). "Hippocrates cancelled," in *Spectator Australia*, 24 October 2020, https://bit.ly/3wED13W.

[412] World Health Organization (2022). Global excess deaths associated with COVID-19, January 2020-December 2021, https://bit.ly/3wK0aAR.

in 2020 than its reported COVID deaths, and no excess deaths in 2021. The WHO report can be seen as prima facie evidence that many of the additional estimated 9 million deaths were caused by lockdowns.

12.4 Estimating the impact on births in Australia

In a previous section (8.3.1) I examined the birth statistics for 2020 released by the ABS (the latest official figures available) and concluded that a net zero estimated effect of lockdowns on births is fair for the purpose of this report.

12.5 Estimating additional non-COVID mortality from lockdowns

In this section I estimate that Australia has experienced **at least 7,940 additional non-COVID deaths due to lockdowns**. I have combined two pieces of data to arrive at this estimate:

- First, longer-term mortality trends in Australia can be used to generate an estimate of counterfactual deaths in 2020 had COVID not emerged. A comparison of actual deaths to forecasts based on these longer-term trends, combined with data on the number of reported COVID deaths, will yield an estimate of additional non-COVID deaths.

- The ABS release on total 2021 deaths is expected on 29 September 2022, in the absence of which provisional mortality reports released by the ABS in 2021 provide information about additional non-COVID deaths.

12.5.1 *Non-COVID deaths in 2020*

Mortality data for Australia since 1915 was released by the ABS on 29 September 2021. Total deaths in recent years are listed in Table 12.1.

2015	159,052
2016	158,504
2017	160,909
2018	158,493
2019	169,301
2020	161,300

Table 12.1: Total deaths in Australia since 2015[413]

The year 2019 is a huge outlier: it seems that deaths in Australia increased by 10,061 in 2019 compared with the average of the previous 4 years (159,240), an increase of 6.3%. This statistical anomaly is partly attributable to the way the ABS counts deaths. Its explanation:

> In 2019, there was an increase of 10,808 deaths compared with the number of deaths registered in 2018. All jurisdictions except the Australian Capital Territory recorded an increase.

> Victoria had the largest increase (5,713 deaths). As a result of joint investigations between the ABS and the Victorian Registry, 2,812 death registrations from 2017, 2018 and 2019 were identified that had not previously been provided to the ABS. Of the 2,812 deaths, 40.4% were registered in 2017, 57.0% in 2018 and the remainder (2.6%) in 2019.

> An issue associated with the Registry's previous processing system (replaced in 2019) resulted in delays to the provision of some death registrations to the ABS. The 2,812 Victorian deaths are in scope of the 2019 reference year and are therefore included in this issue.

> New South Wales recorded the second largest increase (2,425 deaths) which reflected more timely registration of deaths, particularly those that occurred in November and December 2019.[414]

---

[413] Australian Bureau of Statistics (2021). "Deaths, Australia," 29 September 2021, https://bit.ly/3wEDseH.

[414] ABS (2020). "Deaths, Australia methodology, Reference period 2019," 24 September 2020, https://archive.ph/EDvUr.

This information is best read in conjunction with the following description of the methodological processes of the ABS (*ibid*):

> Prior to 2007, the scope for the reference year of the Death Registrations collection included:
>
> - deaths registered in the reference year and received by the ABS in the reference year
> - deaths registered in the reference year and received by the ABS in the first quarter of the subsequent year
> - deaths registered during the two years prior to the reference year but not received by the ABS until the reference year.
>
> From 2007 onwards, the scope for each reference year of the Death Registrations collection includes:
>
> - deaths registered in the reference year and received by the ABS in the reference year
> - deaths registered in the reference year and received by the ABS in the first quarter of the subsequent year
> - deaths registered in the years prior to the reference year but not received by the ABS until the reference year or the first quarter of the subsequent year, provided that these records have not been included in any statistics from earlier periods.

An accurate figure for births and deaths each year is of the greatest policy significance. Arguably, the ABS should produce a corrected or revised table that reports all deaths in the year in which they occurred. In the absence of such a table, from a reading of ABS's footnotes, Table 12.2 is probably closer to the truth:

Year	ABS reference year deaths	Reallocation of Victorian deaths	Actual deaths during the year
2015	159,052		159,052
2016	158,504		158,504
2017	160,909	+1136	162,045
2018	158,493	+1602	160,095
2019	169,301	-2738	166,357
2020	161,300		161,300

Table 12.2: Actual deaths in Australia, 2015-2020, based on interpreting ABS's footnotes

Even with this adjustment, the increase in deaths in 2019 from 2018 by 6,262 is extremely large.

A bad flu year in 2019?

2019's flu season featured sporadic reports of "record numbers of patients flooding into emergency departments,"[415] but overall, according to the Department of Health, the "[c]linical severity for the 2019 season, as measured through the proportion of patients admitted directly to intensive care units (ICU), and deaths attributed to influenza, was moderate."

In 2019, 988 additional deaths were reported from influenza and pneumonia compared with 2018, but it is possible that some of these deaths might have occurred in the previous years. Attributing them all to 2019, these flu deaths would still explain only 16% of the additional 6,262 deaths reported for 2019. There were 956 additional deaths from dementia in 2019, as well as increases in deaths for a wide range of other causes, some of which again might have occurred in previous years, though we cannot be sure.

A year of excess deaths is typically followed by a year of reduced deaths

There is a tendency for more people to die the year following a mild flu year (the "dry tinder" effect, explained earlier as it pertained to

---

[415] *Sydney Morning Herald*. "Flu hits 21,000 people, as NSW hospitals flooded with cases," 14 June 2019, https://archive.ph/E7nfK.

Sweden in 2020), and the reverse is also true: an unusually deadly flu season is typically followed by a season with fewer than usual deaths. More generally, whatever the cause of higher mortality in a given year, high-mortality years are typically followed by years of lower mortality, since fewer vulnerable people are around in the ensuing year to die. Following this logic, one would expect Australia to see a dip in deaths in 2020, to make up for the high mortality of 2019. The amount of this dip would be expected to correspond to the amount by which deaths unexpectedly rose in 2019 – so, in this case, we should expect approximately 6000 fewer deaths in 2020 than what recent trends would forecast. Yet, Table 12.2 shows that the number of deaths in 2020 was quite in line with the numbers of deaths reported in 2017 and 2018. This logic leads to the conclusion that Australia experienced excess deaths in 2020 in the amount of approximately 6000 people.

We also know that COVID basically replaced influenza in the mortality statistics in 2020, with 898 deaths from COVID compared with an average of 626 flu deaths per year over the previous four years, but only double-digit flu deaths in 2020.[416] Hence, these excess deaths were not due to flu, and Australia's COVID deaths were not unusual in number: a similar number of people would have been expected to die of flu in 2020 as died with COVID.

The additional deaths in 2020 beyond what would have been predicted were mainly non-COVID deaths, since fewer than 1000 COVID deaths were recorded that year. Given the growing evidence worldwide of significant loss of life during the pandemic period in locked-down nations,[417] it would be reasonable to interpret these as lockdown-related deaths unless evidence to the contrary is forth-

---

[416] *Source*: NewsGP, "Flu-zero: More than a year since Australia's last flu death," 16 August 2021, https://archive.ph/t7pfl.

[417] The WHO report released on 5 May 2022 is probably the most comprehensive study yet on excess deaths. Combining its information with that from Sweden, this interpretation looks even more likely. (World Health Organization. "14.9 million excess deaths associated with the COVID-19 pandemic in 2020 and 2021," 5 May 2022, https://archive.ph/GylIA).

coming. As illustrated with examples in section 12.3, non-COVID deaths increased in 2020 across the world in nations that adopted lockdowns. Mechanisms for these increases are clear and plausible. For example, within weeks of the March 2020 lockdowns and the hysteria caused by the government, presentations at hospitals and general practices across Australia dropped by around 50% across the board. There were "worrying declines of up to 50% in new cancer patients and 30% in cardiac emergencies, according to Victorian experts."[418]

Some excess deaths might have happened anyway in the counter-factual no-lockdown policy scenario, due to the natural fear of the virus in the population. However, since I have attributed all excess deaths in 2020 in Sweden to COVID, and as there were no excess deaths in Sweden in 2021, the counterfactual no-lockdown non-CO-VID death count in Sweden is likely to be low. Swedes were repeat-edly encouraged by their public health agency to live as normal a life as possible and get themselves treated as usual.[419]

Despite the lack of supporting evidence from an examination of Sweden, I assume conservatively that some of the additional 6,000 reported deaths that were not expected in 2020 in Australia may have happened anyway due to disruptions overseas, even if Australia had pursued a no-lockdown strategy within its borders, because of the interdependence of global markets and communities, plus some amount of COVID fear that could not be reduced via government efforts. I conservatively count 60% of these roughly 6,000 excess deaths in 2020, or **3,600** excess deaths not due to COVID, as **lock-down deaths**.

12.5.2 *Non-COVID excess deaths in 2021*

We have conclusive evidence of additional non-COVID deaths in Australia in 2021. Even using as a comparator the average yearly

---

[418] NewsGP, "Drastic drop in cancer and heart attack patients linked to COVID-19," 14 April 2020, https://bit.ly/3wCIHvz.

[419] Anders Tegnell in a Zoom interview, https://youtu.be/Y2qXJYPQxpU (from the 10-second mark).

deaths in 2015-2019, thus including the outlier year 2019, the provisional mortality data for 2021 that the ABS published in March 2022 (detailed in the sub-section below) indicate that 8,639 excess deaths occurred in Australia in 2021. There were 1,406 reported COVID deaths in Australia during 2021, leaving 7,233 of the excess deaths in 2021 to be counted as non-COVID deaths. Following the same logic as I present above, I conservatively assume that 60% of these deaths, or **4,340 deaths**, were non-COVID lockdown deaths. These deaths were mainly from cancer, dementia, and diabetes.

Combining this figure with the estimate of 3,600 excess non-COVID deaths from 2020, we get a total of **7,940 additional non-COVID deaths from lockdowns in the first two years of the pandemic.**

An analysis of the age distribution of those who died shows that all of these additional 7,940 deaths were of people older than 65 (persons 0-44 (-396 from trend); persons 45-64 (-63), persons 65-74 (+2,029), persons 75-84 (+3,987), persons 85 and over (+4,836). I assume conservatively that the normal care withheld from the average lockdown victim could have potentially saved only 5 years of healthy life for him or her. This assumption enables me to create an estimate of the amount of well-being that these excess deaths caused by lockdowns represent: 7,950 deaths x 5 healthy years= 39,750 QALYs, or **238,500 WELLBYs lost over 2 years**. This translates to **9,937 WELLBYs per month**. This is my estimate of the human well-being that was lost in Australia in 2020 and 2021 due to the immediate effects on mortality of lockdowns.

Australia's excess deaths in 2021: A closer look

On 30 March 2022 the ABS published Provisional Mortality Statistics[420] for the period 4 January 2021 to 2 January 2022. Figure 12.1 is from this data release.

---

[420] Australian Bureau of Statistics. Provisional Mortality Statistics, 30 March 2022, https://archive.ph/Chc3s.

Doctor certified deaths, COVID-19 infections, Australia, 4 Jan 2021 - 2 Jan 2022 vs 2015-2019 benchmarks

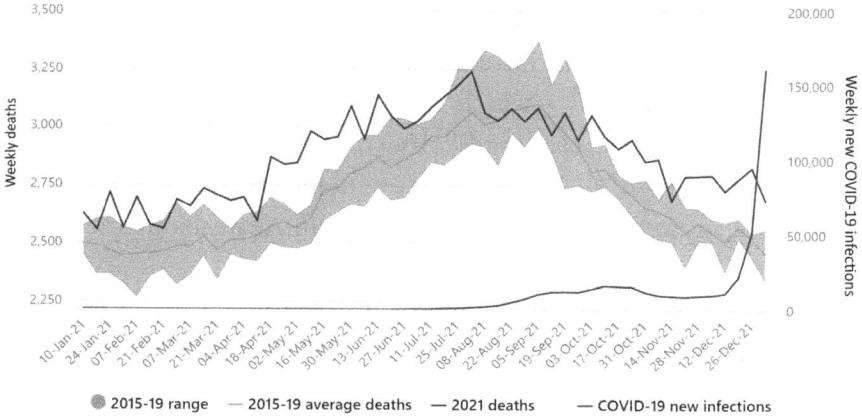

Figure 12.1: Deaths in 2021 compared with the 2015-2019 average
(Source: cited above)

These data suggest that 8,639 excess deaths occurred in Australia in 2021, even including the outlier year of 2019 in generating the expected death count. There were only 1,406 COVID deaths in Australia during this period, so around 7,233 additional deaths (Figure 12.2) are likely to have been caused by Australia's lockdown-based policy response.

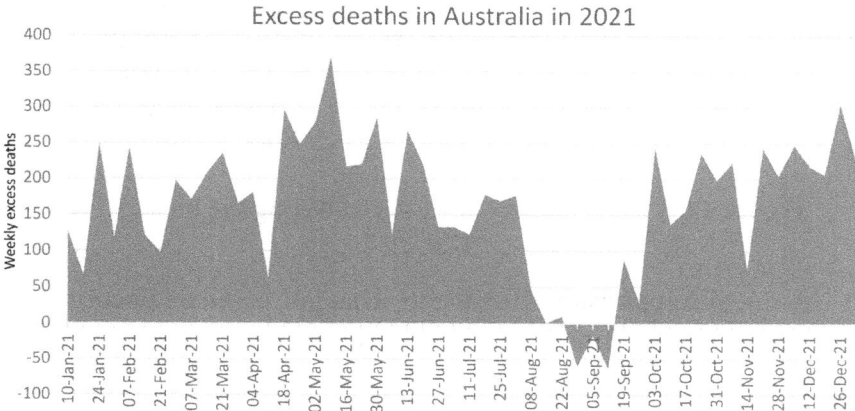

Figure 12.2: Excess deaths in Australia during 2021 (Source: *ibid*)

ABS data suggest that many of these excess deaths are from cancer, diabetes and dementia. There were 3,146 excess cancer deaths in

2021, 1,947 excess dementia deaths and 494 excess diabetes deaths. By contrast, there were 640 fewer deaths related to cerebrovascular diseases (ICD-10 codes I60-I69) such as strokes, carotid stenosis, vertebral stenosis and intracranial stenosis, aneurysms, and vascular malformations – which could be caused by known vaccine side effects such as clotting.[421] Together with Sweden's lack of excess mortality in 2021, this is some evidence that COVID vaccines had not caused noticeable excess deaths in Australia by the end of 2021.

Was there a small reduction in deaths during lockdowns in early 2020?

While I have estimated 3,600 excess non-COVID deaths for 2020, Figure 12.3 suggests a small reduction in overall deaths may have occurred during the first few months of lockdowns.

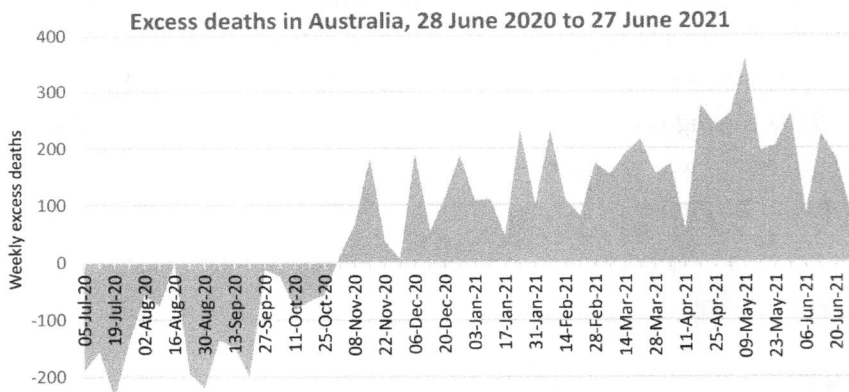

Excess deaths in Australia, 28 June 2020 to 27 June 2021

Figure 12.3: Excess deaths in Australia during the financial year 2020-21[422]

This visual comparison of fortnightly changes, based on uncorrected March 2022 ABS data which does not exclude the outlier year 2019

---

[421] E.g., Sun, Christopher L.F. et al (2022). "Increased emergency cardiovascular events among under-40 population in Israel during vaccine rollout and third COVID-19 wave," *Scientific Reports*, 12:6978, https://doi.org/10.1038/s41598-022-10928-z, https://www.nature.com/articles/s41598-022-10928-z.pdf.

[422] Spreadsheet at https://bit.ly/3NHiKkh. *Source data*: Australian Bureau of Statistics. Provisional Mortality Statistics, 30 March 2022, https://archive.ph/Chc3s.

from the figures used as comparators, indicates an initial reduction in deaths that may be due to the exceptionally high reported deaths in 2019. Could it also be possible that initially, lockdowns were not causing excess deaths, and in fact were preventing them?

The potential positive impacts on death counts from lowered homicides and lower traffic fatalities during lockdowns have already been considered and incorporated into the Benefits chapter of this report. Also, in the normal course of events, when we close hospitals, deaths are indeed reduced in the short run. This is because hospitals perform many surgeries that improve quality of life, like hip replacements, knee surgery, organ transplantations, and so on, and these surgeries all carry a small additional risk of immediate death. When these services are shut down, death counts from such surgeries fall.

In COVID times, even high-risk patients were denied surgeries and presented less frequently to emergency rooms. Ambulance calls dropped (000 calls dropped by 30% in Victoria, for example[423]). While some of these non-calls may have led to deaths due to lack of immediate treatment, many of those denied immediate treatment will have pulled through for a few more months and died later.

In the UK, deaths at home rose almost immediately after lockdowns were imposed.[424] According to a chart published in Yahoo News, excess deaths at home in the UK in 2020 followed a steady upward trend starting 15 days into lockdowns. Therefore, while the elective surgery effect might have dominated the excess deaths data during the first two weeks, it seems to have been swamped quickly by the overall negative effects of lockdowns on care. ONS data further show that only 8,824 – or 12% – of 75,474 excess deaths in the UK during 2020 involved COVID.[425]

---

[423] *The Age.* "Triple-zero calls drop in Victoria, but paramedics brace for surge," 19 April 2020, https://bit.ly/3Nswdw4.

[424] *Source: Yahoo News.* "More than 75,000 extra deaths at home in England and Wales since pandemic began," 9 November 2021, https://archive.ph/mBwpX.

[425] *Source:* Office for National Statistics. "Deaths at home increased by a third in 2020, while deaths in hospitals fell except for COVID-19," 7 May 2021, https://archive.ph/Hivm6.

Further additional deaths from cancers and other diseases that were not detected in the early stages of lockdowns will take time to manifest, and some of these will have appeared in the 2021 data.

12.5.3 *Excess deaths in 2021: Comparing Australia and Sweden*

As noted above, Sweden experienced a significant decline in total deaths during 2021 compared to previous years. Its overall mortality rate for 2021, at 88.3 out of 10,000, is close to the lowest in its history,[426] and it is the lowest when adjusting for the dry tinder effect of 2019.

Figure 12.4 compares the excess deaths in Australia (not adjusting for the 2019 outlier) and in Sweden in 2021. The figure supports the argument that Australia's surge in non-COVID deaths is likely attributable to its lockdowns, which Sweden avoided.

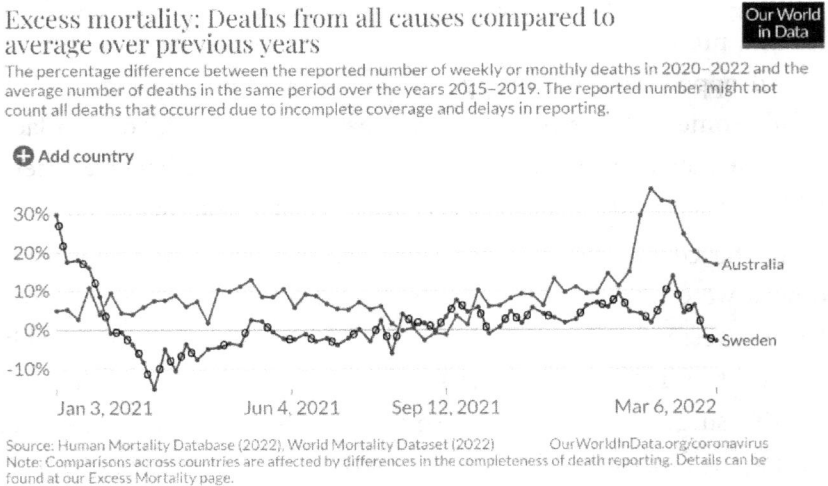

Excess mortality: Deaths from all causes compared to average over previous years

Our World in Data

The percentage difference between the reported number of weekly or monthly deaths in 2020–2022 and the average number of deaths in the same period over the years 2015–2019. The reported number might not count all deaths that occurred due to incomplete coverage and delays in reporting.

Source: Human Mortality Database (2022), World Mortality Dataset (2022)   OurWorldInData.org/coronavirus
Note: Comparisons across countries are affected by differences in the completeness of death reporting. Details can be found at our Excess Mortality page.

Figure 12.4: Excess mortality since January 2021 – comparison of Australia and Sweden[427]

---

[426] Statistics Sweden (SCB). "Mortality rate per 1,000 of the mean population by age and sex. Year 2000-2020," https://bit.ly/3MEgmdX.

[427] *Source*: Our World in Data. Excess Mortality: Deaths from all causes compared to average over previous years, Sweden and Australia, 2021, https://bit.ly/38IyTHb. Also see the analysis of excess deaths by independent researcher Jose Gefaell at https://bit.ly/3wDoBRF.

12.5.4 *Excess deaths in the UK*

Euromomo has produced charts depicting the annual excess deaths of various European nations.[428] Data on the UK's excess deaths from 2019 through 2022 suggests that the "dry tinder" effect that affected Sweden in 2019 may have also operated on the UK, priming the country for more deaths in 2020. The death rates for 2020 in the UK, which imposed stringent lockdowns, are still higher than Sweden's.[429]

Figure 12.5, taken from a 16 November 2021 report in *The Telegraph*,[430] confirms the pattern of excess deaths in the UK. The report noted that "9,292 deaths – 45 per cent – were not linked to the pandemic" (meaning, not involving COVID).

Total deaths from all causes
Number of deaths registered in England and Wales by week ending

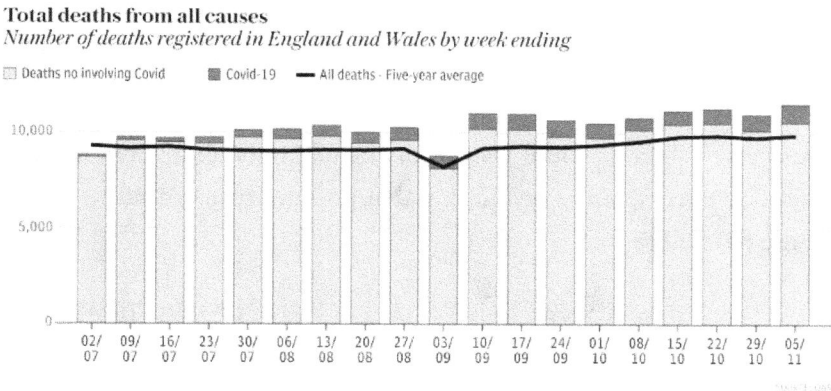

Figure 12.5: Total deaths in England and Wales by week, July-November 2021

Unlike in Australia, it seems excess deaths occurred in 2021 even in the 0-65 age group in the UK. Nobel Prize-winning scientist Michael Levitt noted on 12 November 2021 that:

> UK England & Wales had 27% excess under 65. Was the same price paid in Sweden? No way as no excess deaths under or over 65 years old. What about the USA? Will be even

---

[428] *Source:* Euromomo, https://archive.ph/rongv.

[429] Tweet dated 19 August 2021 by Anthony Sargeant, https://archive.ph/YhOCy.

[430] *The Telegraph* (2021). "Alarm grows as mortuaries fill with thousands of extra non-Covid deaths," 16 November 2021, https://archive.ph/jI26H.

worse than UK as excess deaths under 65 are 37%, a percentage still rising.[431]

12.5.5 *Excess deaths elsewhere in the world in 2021*

In the US, there is evidence[432] of excess deaths in the 25-65 age group evenly distributed across the months of 2020 and 2021 compared with the stand-out peaks that largely consisted of COVID deaths. This suggests the policy response, rather than the virus itself, as the cause of these excess deaths amongst people younger than the average COVID victim.

Other countries that locked down have also reported significant increases in excess non-COVID deaths (e.g., Ireland, reporting around 200 excess non-COVID deaths per month[433]). The WHO's May 2022 report[434] identified 14.9 million excess deaths globally between 1 January 2020 and 31 December 2021, despite only 5.42 million of these being reported as COVID deaths. Some fraction of these excess deaths could potentially be attributable to COVID vaccine side effects, but investigating that possibility is out of the scope of the current report.

12.6 Opportunity cost: Deaths that could have been avoided with a different expenditure of COVID dollars

According to the Australian Institute of Health and Welfare:

> Potentially avoidable deaths are deaths among people younger than 75 that are potentially avoidable within the present health care system. They include deaths from conditions that are potentially preventable through individualised care and/or treatable through existing primary or hospital care. In 2019, there were 28,000 potentially avoidable

---

[431] Tweet dated 11 November 2021 by Michael Levitt, https://bit.ly/38LHIzT.

[432] *Source*: Tweet dated 4 October 2021 by Ben@USMortality, https://archive.ph/pWV66.

[433] *Business Post*. "Data from funeral site shows sharp rise in excess deaths in recent months," 7 November 2021, https://bit.ly/3MFm9zD.

[434] World Health Organization, "14.9 million excess deaths associated with the COVID-19 pandemic in 2020 and 2021," 5 May 2022, https://archive.ph/GylIA.

deaths: half (48%) of all deaths for people aged less than 75. Of these deaths, 64% were male and 36% were female.[435]

An estimate could be made of how many lives could have been saved if the hundreds of billions of dollars spent by the government on lockdowns had instead been directed towards other health priorities. That number of lives potentially saved would represent the opportunity cost of Australia's COVID policy response. Arguably, thousands of non-COVID deaths could have been avoided in 2020 and 2021 with the vast sums of money spent on postponing COVID deaths allegedly through lockdowns and the expenditures made to cushion their fallout.

12.7 Estimating the effects of lockdowns on lifespan

The long-term adverse health effects from lockdowns of increased obesity, increased substance abuse, reduced immunity from reduced social connections and support, disrupted education of children, and a medium-term increase in health problems like cancer, are likely to have a small but ultimately measurable effect on the lives of all Australians.

a) Long-term effects of increased obesity

The increase in obesity in Australia in 2020 and 2021 would have made some people more vulnerable to COVID itself. Yet more generally, obesity has been shown to have long-term impacts on mortality.[436] Xu et al (2018) observe that it is not just obesity at the time of death, but having been obese earlier in life, that carries a longevity cost: "The mortality rates of normal-weight individuals who were

---

[435] Australian Institute of Health and Welfare. "Deaths in Australia," 25 June 2021, https://bit.ly/3wzA2tG.

[436] Xu, Hanfei et al (2018). "Association of Obesity With Mortality Over 24 Years of Weight History," in *JAMA Netw Open,*;1(7):e184587. doi:10.1001/jamanetworkopen.2018.4587, https://jamanetwork.com/journals/jamanetworkopen/fullarticle/2714501; also see a 2018 report (Tobias, Deirdre K. et al (2018), "The association between BMI and mortality: implications for obesity prevention," in *The Lancet Diabetes and Endocrinology*, Volume 6, Issue 12, pp. 916-917, 1 December 2018) that discusses "the strong association between increasing BMI and excess mortality," based on studies of 3.6 million adults in the UK (https://www.thelancet.com/journals/landia/article/PIIS2213-8587(18)30309-7/fulltext).

formerly overweight or obese were 47.48 and 66.67 per 1000 person-years, respectively, while individuals who never exceeded normal weight had a mortality rate of 27.93 per 1000 person-years."

A report by the organisation AUSActive notes that "[m]odelling by Deakin University Health Economics found that the 25% drop in physical activity levels due to COVID-19 will add a $1.5 billion burden to the healthcare system, even if levels return to normal by April 2022."[437]

How soon will people revert to their old exercise habits? Many people may have resumed their gym memberships in 2022, but the combination of mental health harms experienced from lockdowns, reduced long-term earning capacity through lost skills or early unplanned retirement, and sheer inertia could see a small but significant proportion of the population unable to lose the weight and poor health habits taken on during lockdowns. The trend of working from home, precipitated by lockdowns but still continuing, may also reduce levels of everyday exercise like walking during commutes.

b) Medium-term increase in cancers

As discussed earlier, many cancers were not identified and treated in time during lockdowns. While increased cancer deaths are already visible in the mortality statistics for 2021, this effect is likely to continue for another year or two. Habits developed during lockdowns such as increased consumption of fast foods and processed foods – excess consumption of which is known to cause cancer – are also likely to precipitate more cancers in the coming years.[438]

c) Long-term harms from alcohol and substance abuse

Alcohol and drugs are addictive, so it is possible that some of those who increased their intake of substances during lockdowns will go on to develop a lifelong habit that can cause other harms. The WHO estimates that "Overall, 5.1% of the global burden of disease and in-

[437] AUSActive. "A more active Australia for a healthier nation: Research and economic modelling into physical inactivity and COVID-19," https://bit.ly/3lNUGQJ.
[438] Cancer Council. "Red meat, processed meat and cancer," https://archive.ph/bxwD7.

jury is attributable to alcohol, as measured in disability-adjusted life years (DALYs)."[439] The precise magnitude of any longer-term change in alcohol and drug habits in Australia resulting from lockdowns will take time to determine.

How does one estimate these long-term effects? Evidence from other nations indicates that measurable long-term health impacts of lockdowns on the general population are a real possibility.

- A 12 November 2020 paper that limited its scope to estimating the impact of school closures on life expectancy concluded that: "missed instruction during 2020 could be associated with an estimated 13.8 (95% CI 2.5-42.1) million years of life lost based on data from US studies and an estimated 0.8 (95% CI 0.1-2.4) million years of life lost based on data from European studies."[440]

- A December 2020 NBER working paper, revised in September 2021, considers the long-term mortality impact of the COVID unemployment shock (caused by both COVID itself and the policy response) in the US and concludes that more than 0.8 million additional deaths will occur over the next 15 years as a result.[441] The paper does not consider the longevity effect of a host of other impacts of lockdowns.

- A December 2020 study concluded that lockdowns in Indonesia had "reduced life expectancy by up to 1.7 years."[442]

In Australia, the government provided financial compensation during lockdowns that may have acted to stem some longevity effects of lockdowns, but not all such effects can be negated with monetary

---

[439] World Health Organization. Alcohol. 21 September 2018, https://archive.ph/EQNPv.

[440] Christakis, Dimitri A. et al (2020). "Estimation of US Children's Educational Attainment and Years of Life Lost Associated With Primary School Closures During the Coronavirus Disease 2019 Pandemic," in *JAMA Network Open*; 3(11):e2028786. doi:10.1001/jamanetworkopen.2020.28786, https://jamanetwork.com/journals/jamanetworkopen/fullarticle/2772834.

[441] Bianchi, Francesco et al (2021), "The Long-Term Impact Of The Covid-19 Unemployment Shock On Life Expectancy And Mortality Rates," NBER Working Paper 28304, https://www.nber.org/system/files/working_papers/w28304/w28304.pdf.

[442] Gibson, John et al (2020). "Direct and Indirect Effects of Covid-19 On Life Expectancy and Poverty in Indonesia," in *Bulletin of Indonesian Economic Studies*, 4 Dec 2020, pp. 325-344, https://www.tandfonline.com/eprint/73TNAMP7JXVBVYYYFYWG/full.

handouts. Given the uncertainty of the magnitude of these less-visible harms, but fairly strong preliminary evidence of their existence, I include a conservative, long-term residual negative effect of lockdowns on overall mortality over and above what is included in my estimates for other cost categories. It can be argued that there is some overlap in this discussion of health harms with the harms to well-being that are discussed and quantified already, but I assume that these latter effects will stop after 2021, whereas the effects being considered in this section are those that will spill into the future and are therefore not captured elsewhere in this report.

Very conservatively, I assume that in addition to other harms, lockdowns will reduce by one week on average berween the remaining lifespan of each Australian who lived through lockdowns.

This yields 25.7/52 million QALYs, or a total of **494,230 QALYs** lost. These losses will manifest over the remainder of our lives. Limiting this tail of future losses to a span of 50 years,[443] this translates to 9,884 QALYs lost per year, or **59,304** WELLBYs lost per year for the next 50 years, or **4,942 WELLBYs lost per month** in Australia for the next 50 years.

---

[443] Theoretically, this 50-year estimate is a conservative, crude approximation, because the babies born during lockdowns will be expected to live for 80+ years, meaning that lifespan reductions due to lockdowns will continue beyond a 50-year window. A complex calculation based on age structure would be needed to refine this estimate. For the final calculation of cost impact, I discount future costs like this by 5%, but on that issue as well there can be many refinements.

13. Mostly future costs: (4) Sustained damage to productivity

Lockdowns may cause the following effects on Australian productivity:

a) loss of productivity among today's youth, the employed, and entrepreneurs; and

b) loss of productivity among today's children once they reach adulthood.

13.1 Longer-term productivity impacts of lockdowns on the young, employed, and entrepreneurs

Longer-term productivity costs to society in this category are likely non-zero, but I make the conservative choice of omitting them from my estimates of the harms of lockdowns. I sketch these sorts of effects below for completeness.

13.1.1 *Reduction in training for the young*

Lockdowns adversely affected the formal training of apprentices and young workers in Australia.[444] A reduction in learning within organisations, particularly for new recruits, is also likely due to reductions in learning-by-doing and observing experts. Unplanned "water-cooler" conversations in corridors and lifts, in which productive links are formed and the informal insights of experienced workers are shared, are vitally important for young workers. These interactions cannot be replicated in an online work environment.

This loss of quality training for young workers across Australia for two years will likely have lifelong impacts on their productivity and earning capacity.

---

[444] "There was a steep rise in contract suspensions in March, April and May. Another spike occurred in August as Victoria endured its lengthy second lockdown through the winter." *Source*: AI Group (2021). "Pandemic impact on apprenticeships: NCVER data," 24 September 2021, https://archive.ph/VErtf.

13.1.2 *Reduced opportunities for leadership development*

Lockdowns are likely to have reduced the leadership capability of the COVID cohort of youth, due to reduced workplace training as discussed above but also for other reasons. Active participation in sports, arts, music, and community activities develop skills that future leaders need. The reduction in social and sporting events during lockdowns is likely to have a long-term negative impact on the social skills of the young, including a reduction in their capability as leaders.

13.1.3 *Loss of initiative and the desire to participate and produce*

The observation that government can destroy the efforts of entrepreneurs in the blink of an eye could lead overall to a reduced desire to produce. Lockdowns have signalled clearly to producers that the government has the power to disable citizens' physical movements and confiscate not just their right to work, but their business and property rights. Some former employees and entrepreneurs are looking to escape what mainstream life has become by going "off-grid," with a reported 77% increase in real estate searches for "off-grid" properties.[445]

On the other hand, as mentioned earlier, there might have been some countervailing benefits of lockdowns on productivity, due for example to an accelerated shift towards automation and newly discovered applications of online technology.

13.2 Reduced investment by domestic and foreign investors

Mass-scale protests in several Australian capital cities against lockdowns and vaccine mandates, and the poor performance of both major parties in the May 2022 elections (Liberal and Labor both polled first-preference votes at or close to the lowest in their history), indicate growing malaise in the Australian community.

Civil unrest and a perceived loss of confidence in Australian lead-

---

[445] Realestate.com (2021). "More Aussie house hunters looking to go 'off grid' in COVID's wake," 24 February 2021, https://archive.ph/vx8IO.

ership may impact the decisions of investors at home and overseas, which would in turn reduce longer-run productivity growth. On the other hand, investors tend to be agnostic and are likely to invest wherever they sense an opportunity for upside gain, which may well be when things look bleak. I therefore ignore this possible longer-term impact on investment.

13.3 Lifetime reduction in productivity of children born during lockdowns

It takes a village to grow a bright, happy, healthy child. Lockdowns damaged the normal functioning of families and communities that nurture children in normal times, and through these means, lockdowns damaged children.

The latest data indicates that lost socialisation of infants during lockdowns has had a measurable and exceptionally strong negative effect on intelligence. While summarising a study by Deoni et al[446] as "news," the *BMJ* reported on 16 August 2021 that:

> In a longitudinal study of 672 children from Rhode Island that has run since 2011, those born after the pandemic began showed results on the Mullen scales of early learning that corresponded to an average IQ score of 78, a drop of 22 points from the average of previous cohorts.[447]

This effect is attributed to "reduced interaction with parents and less outdoor exercise … along with effects that occurred during pregnancy." The Deoni et al study (awaiting publication, reportedly in *JAMA Pediatrics,* at the time of writing) notes that during the lockdowns:

> [f]ear of infection and possible employment loss has placed stress on parents; while parents who could work from

---

[446] Deoni, Sean C.L. et al (2021). "Impact of the COVID-19 Pandemic on Early Child Cognitive Development: Initial Findings in a Longitudinal Observational Study of Child Health," in *medRxiv,* 2021.08.10.21261846. https://doi.org/10.1101/2021.08.10.21261846 (awaiting publication in *JAMA Paediatrics*).

[447] Dyer, Owen (2021). "Covid-19: Children born during the pandemic score lower on cognitive tests, study finds," in *BMJ* 2021; 374, published 16 August 2021, https://www.bmj.com/content/374/bmj.n2031.

home faced challenges in both working and providing full-time attentive childcare. For pregnant individuals, fear of attending prenatal visits also increased maternal stress, anxiety, and depression. Not surprising, there has been concern over how these factors, as well as missed educational opportunities and reduced interaction, stimulation, and creative play with other children might impact child neurodevelopment. Leveraging a large on-going longitudinal study of child neurodevelopment, we examined general childhood cognitive scores in 2020 and 2021 vs. the preceding decade, 2011-2019. We find that children born during the pandemic have significantly reduced verbal, motor, and overall cognitive performance compared to children born pre-pandemic. Moreover, we find that males and children in lower socioeconomic families have been most affected.

This effect seems to be limited to a small group of children, since "[c]hildren born in 2019 did not experience a decline in development scores during the pandemic ... Their trajectories of maturation were unaltered ... They seemed to be doing alright. It's really affecting those born during the pandemic, whether through transference from their mother, what she's experiencing during late term pregnancy, or during those crucial earliest months after birth."

Masking policies are likely to have played a role. The "Still Face" experiment conducted by researchers at the University of Massachusetts Boston in 2009 found that prolonged situations of not seeing a responsive face of a person can make a child become disoriented.[448] A video is available.[449]

While the Deoni et al study is from Rhode Island in the US, and is not peer-reviewed at the time of writing, there could be implications for at least some of the roughly 600,000 children born during 2020 and 2021 in Australia. Is there any supporting evidence? The *BMJ*

---

[448] Tweet dated 5 October 2021 by Erich Hartman, https://archive.ph/o1WUQ.
[449] http://youtu.be/vmE3NfB_HhE.

"news" reporting of 16 August 2021, referred to above, notes that: "Other research has hinted at behavioural effects in children born during the pandemic, including a recent study from Italy"[450] – which is cited.

Some loss in IQ, if it occurs in Australian children, may be reversible with education, but it seems unlikely that losses can be completely reversed given the short window of developmental opportunity presented in early childhood. Assuming conservatively that the IQ of 0.6 million Australian children drops permanently by only a few points on average, this would have a significant impact on future productivity and wages.

Impact of IQ on future earnings

While the concept that IQ will correlate with future earnings seems intuitive, it is difficult to pin down an estimate of this effect that is free from contamination by social, cultural and economic factors. For example, SAT scores in the US have been found to correlate more with a family's prior wealth than with the scorer's future earnings (which might indicate the genetic transmission of intelligence, or that the ability to fund preparation for the SAT exams is important).[451]

Angrist and Krueger's famous 1991 study of future earnings payoffs from schooling[452] controlled for ability using the Armed Forces Qualification Test (AFQT) score (IQ scores were not available). Future earnings are also highly related to personality traits,[453] meaning that many highly intelligent individuals do not earn more than oth-

[450] Dyer, Owen (2021). "Covid-19: Children born during the pandemic score lower on cognitive tests, study finds," in *BMJ* 2021; 374 doi: https://doi.org/10.1136/bmj.n2031, published 16 August 2021, https://www.bmj.com/content/374/bmj.n2031.

[451] Sandel, Michael J. (2020). "High family income, not SAT scores, is your real ticket to Harvard, Yale, and Princeton," in *ThePrint*, 19 November 2020, https://archive.ph/v2jmG.

[452] Angrist, Joshua D., and Alan B. Krueger (1991). "Does Compulsory School Attendance Affect Schooling and Earnings?" in *The Quarterly Journal of Economics* 106, no. 4 (1991): 979–1014, https://doi.org/10.2307/2937954.

[453] Gensowski, Miriam (2014). "Personality, IQ, and Lifetime Earnings," IZA DP No. 8235, June 2014, https://ftp.iza.org/dp8235.pdf.

ers, either because they do not want to earn more or because their personality gets in the way.

It has been suggested that high school scores are a better predictor of innate intelligence and do not suffer as much as other measures do from contamination by economic or social factors.[454] Figure 13.1, based on a 2014 article published in the *Eastern Economic Journal*,[455] shows a fairly robust relationship between high school grade point average (a proxy for intelligence) and earnings.

Average annual earnings in adulthood, by high school GPA

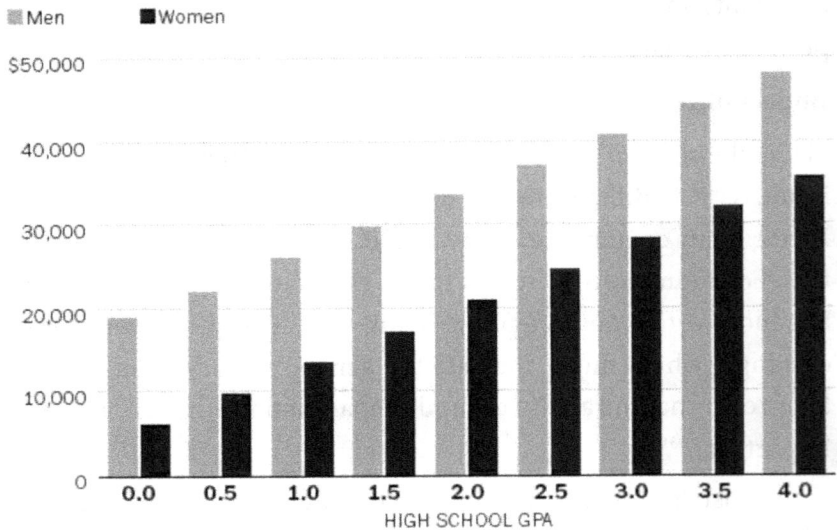

SOURCE: University of Miami
GRAPHIC: The Washington Post. Published May 20, 2014

Figure 13.1: Relationship between high school GPA and earnings in adulthood

Assuming that the lifetime earnings of each of the 600,000 Australian children born in 2020 and 2021 will drop by even $30,000 (i.e., by

[454] Marte, Jonnelle (2014). "Here's how much your high school grades predict your future salary," in *The Washington Post*, 20 May 2014, https://archive.ph/7GNtP.
[455] French, Michael T., Jenny F. Homer, Ioana Popovici, and Philip K. Robins (2015). "What You Do in High School Matters: High School GPA, Educational Attainment, and Labor Market Earnings as a Young Adult," in *Eastern Economic Journal* 41, no. 3 (2015): 370–86. http://www.jstor.org/stable/24693733. The figure is from *The Washington Post*: https://archive.ph/7GNtP.

just $1,000 per year of work), we recover an estimated total loss of **$18 billion** on average. If as previously argued $100,000 purchases 1 QALY, this yields a loss of 180,000 QALYs over the working lifetimes of these children, or **1,080,000** WELLBYs if these losses manifest as life-years saved.[456] Equivalently, this is 30,857 WELLBYs per year for 35 years. This effect will be observed only after these children enter the workforce.

13.4 Lifetime reduction in productivity from disrupted schooling

In mid-March 2020, a tendency arose in Australia for schools to be closed and students to be transitioned to online learning without any detailed risk-based argument or analysis of the costs and benefits of such a switch.

An analysis by the Public Health Agency of Sweden (which kept schools open for all children under 16) in June 2020 showed no statistical difference in paediatric COVID cases between Sweden and Finland, and no increased risk to teachers compared to other professions.[457] Table 13.1 shows that just 2 children had died with COVID through November 2020 in Sweden. Statista shows a total of 24 reported deaths from COVID of children below the age of 19 through 20 July 2022 in Sweden.[458] Data from various countries confirms that very few of these children are likely to have died directly from COVID, as most had serious co-morbidities.

---

[456] The translation of 1 QALY = 6 WELLBYs only holds when the QALY is manifest in life-years rather than health quality. If only health quality is affected, but not life-years, then a reduction in 1 QALY translates to a reduction in fewer than 6 WELLBYs because other factors apart from health quality affect life satisfaction. Future analysis may refine the estimates here accordingly.

[457] Public Health Agency of Sweden (2020). Covid-19 in schoolchildren: A comparison between Finland and Sweden, https://bit.ly/3MTJ1vI.

[458] Statista. "Number of coronavirus (COVID-19) deaths in Sweden, by age groups," as of 20 July 2022, https://bit.ly/3cJHzPa.

Age group	Cases	Percentage of cases (n=137,730)	Deaths	Proportion of deaths (n=5,997)
0-9	1,107	0.80%	2	0.0%
10-19	9,338	6.80%	0	0.0%
20-29	25,831	18.80%	11	0.2%
30-39	22,778	16.50%	17	0.3%
40-49	23,110	16.80%	46	0.8%
50-59	23,325	16.90%	166	2.8%
60-69	12,808	9.30%	415	6.9%
70-79	7,682	5.60%	1,279	21.3%
80-89	7,655	5.60%	2,491	41.5%
90+	4,071	3.00%	1,570	26.2%

Table 13.1: Number of diagnosed cases of COVID-19 per age group and proportion of total cases and number of deaths (Sweden, as of 5 November 2020)[459]

The effects of lockdowns on children via school closures and associated migration to online education from home are significant and long-lasting. Disruption to children's schooling is known to cause a significant reduction in the future wages of those children. Other effects are also sure to occur, such as higher levels of domestic violence, reduced social skills, and the development of bad habits. When children stay home from school, their learning suffers even as their parents' productivity suffers. Ari Joffe has noted that "[e]arly primary grades are most vulnerable, with effects into adulthood: effects on outcomes of intelligence, teen pregnancy, illicit drug use, graduation rates, employment rates and earnings, arrest rates, hypertension, diabetes mellites, depression."[460]

Professor Ellen Townsend of the Self-Harm Research Group at the University of Nottingham made a submission to the UK Parliament on 10 January 2021 noting:

---

[459] *Source*: Swedish Public Health Agency (2020). "COVID-19 in children and adolescents: A knowledge summary – Version 2," https://bit.ly/3wPIyDZ.

[460] https://www.frontiersin.org/articles/10.3389/fpubh.2021.625778/full, Joffe, A. (2021). "COVID-19: Rethinking the Lockdown Groupthink," in *Frontiers in Public Health*, 9, 98. fpubh.2021.625778.

The impact of school closures owing to lockdowns has been enormous with many missed months of education leading to a regression in basic skills which is fuelling an ever-increasing attainment gap. Missing out on school is life limiting: a study in the US has estimated that 5.53 million Years of Life Lost will be caused by school closures – life expectancies will be affected.[461]

ICAN, a UK organisation, reported in October 2021:

Children learn to speak and understand language through their interactions with others. Covid has massively reduced the amount of social interaction that children of all ages have had over the past two years. It has also reduced the things that children learn to talk about. Without trips out of the classroom or new experiences, there is less reason for children to speak or use new words. Children in deprived areas are particularly at risk – levelling-up cannot happen without children's speaking and understanding being improved.

Children who experience difficulties with speaking and understanding are over four times less likely to pass GCSEs in Maths and English. This can lead to fewer job opportunities, as good communication is rated by employers as the most important skill for young people entering their first job. Indeed, it has been found that 88% of long-term unemployed young men have difficulties with speaking and understanding language.[462]

A November 2021 report in *USA Today* noted that first graders were far behind in reading, and that according to experts these children may take years to catch up.[463]

In a peer-reviewed paper in 2020,[464] I used Australian data from

---

[461] Written evidence from Professor Ellen Townsend (CIL0977), UK Parliament, https://bit.ly/3wHIbv8.

[462] ICAN. "Speaking Up for the Covid Generation," https://bit.ly/3yUtuHO.

[463] *USA Today News.* "Pandemic first graders are way behind in reading. Experts say they may take years to catch up," 14 November 2021, https://archive.ph/yM9cv.

[464] Foster, Gigi (2020). "Early estimates of the impact of COVID-19 disruptions on jobs, wages, and lifetime earnings of schoolchildren in Australia," in *Australian Journal of Labour Economics*, Vol 23 No. 2, https://archive.ph/gX4RT.

the period 14 March to 30 May 2020 to assess the impact on the adult wages of today's schoolchildren whose education has been disrupted due to school closures. My paper targeted the cumulative costs but was limited only to estimates of these children's lifetime earnings foregone. I left out many cost categories affected by school closures, such as:

- the impact of delays in learning to socialise;
- the impact on learning a range of soft skills that make for happier, successful citizens; and
- the longer-run health costs from the loss of the physical activity and exercise in school.

I also made the conservative assumption that online learning is 90% as effective as in-person learning.

Looking only at the cost of children's online rather than face-to-face learning in terms of foregone wages, I estimated that the lifetime wages (which reflect productivity) of Australian schoolchildren denied normal schooling for 2 ½ months in 2020 are on the order of $50-$100 million.

It has not yet been feasible to update the entire list of closures of schools across Australia,[465] but we know that lockdowns continued until well into 2021 in Australia. We also know that school closures intensified after the first 2.5 months.[466] For example, while the rule from 7 April 2020 in Victoria was that "During Term 2 all children who can learn at home must learn from home," from 12 July 2021 it became mandatory for pupils from Prep through Year 10 in metropolitan Melbourne and Mitchell Shire to switch entirely to remote learning.

Assuming that school closures in the first 2.5 months of the COVID era were broadly replicated for another 13 months (excluding

---

[465] The OxCGRT project of the Oxford University is currently building a sub-national database for Australia that includes a field for the severity of school closures.

[466] Parliament of Victoria. "Primary and secondary school closures in Victoria due to COVID-19," https://bit.ly/3Nvdose.

normal school holidays) through 22 October 2021, when Melbourne finally came out of its lockdowns, we recover an estimate of **$465 million** in lost earnings over a 35-year working life,[467] again using the conservative assumption that online learning was 90% as effective as in-person learning.

Assuming that $100,000 buys one QALY, this cost represents the cost of saving 4,650 QALYs, or **27,900 WELLBYs** over 35 years if considered in terms of life-years saved, or (recalling that a COVID death on average represents a sacrifice of 5 QALYs) **930 lives lost of the type typically lost to COVID, in the form of foregone wages of children** who have suffered disrupted schooling during lockdowns.

---

[467] The calculation for the additional 13 months: (13/2.5) x 75 = 390. $75 million is used as it is the mid-point of the $50-$100 million estimate for the 2.5-month cost. To this $390 million we add the initial 2.5-month cost of $75 million to yield $465 million in all.

14. Other costs: (5) Lost social capital, increased crime

In this chapter I discuss some of the many other costs of lockdowns, such as the loss of social capital, longer-term impacts on immigration, and effects on crime and the environment. However, given a lack of robust measures of these costs, I will not estimate them for the purposes of this CBA. Any future CBA of Australia's COVID policy response should re-consider estimating these costs.

14.1 Loss of social capital

Many signs indicate that the social fabric of Australia has been damaged by lockdown policies.[468] The following first-hand anecdote was shared on 3 October 2021 with Sanjeev Sabhlok on social media:

> People are now afraid of interacting with other people. We have relocated to a small rural town that was a hive of creative activity pre COVID. It was known for its artistic events, cultural activities i.e. literature and film, Italian farming community and on a gourmet food trail. That's all on hold. People don't interact out in the streets, avoid eye contact and maintain a level of distance. What was a strong cohesive community is being destroyed by the constant barrage of fear. The community used to welcome and embrace new residents and families, especially the new infants, and support the elderly by monitoring and assisting them but that has been diminished as well. There is a change in the way we live as a human collective and how societies form.[469]

Within formerly close-knit communities and even within families, there has also been significant conflict and difference of opin-

---

[468] E.g., http://youtu.be/emCXhtIm2-U.

[469] Sabhlokcity.com (2022). "An anecdote about how the social fabric of Australia has been torn asunder by totalitarian policies," 1 June 2022, https://archive.ph/eTlKD.

ion about COVID issues and policies, leading in some cases to harsh language being used against those who may not agree with a particular view. Many relationships have been permanently damaged.[470]

A sense of community is crucial to the success of a society. Social capital contributes to a society's overall economic success and mental well-being. The loss of trust, the (sometimes permanent) loss of commercial and personal relationships, and the increased friction in society all necessarily impose costs. These costs overlap to some degree with the mental health costs discussed earlier, but there are also impacts of losses in these intangible realms on productivity, innovation, and the ability to retain people in Australia.

Estimating the loss of Australia's social capital would benefit from specific calibrated surveys. Illustrative work in Australia to measure and assess social capital includes:

- P. Bullen's 1998 "Measuring social capital in five communities in NSW."[471]

- The ABS's 2004 "Information Paper: Measuring Social Capital – An Australian Framework and Indicators."[472]

- The Household Income and Labour Dynamics in Australia (HILDA) survey includes a measure of social support, but its data are slow to be released and an analysis of the impacts of lockdowns is not currently available. However, based on Waves 14 and 15 (July 2014 to Feb 2016) of the HILDA survey, a 2020 Australian study reported that:

> the structural dimension of social capital would function as a buffer against the malicious effects of chronic health

---

[470] Hu, Jane (2021). "What Did COVID Do to Friendship?" in *The New Yorker*, 11 June 2021, https://archive.ph/CqGlY; Dastagir, Alia (2021). "Siblings fighting. Spouses at odds. How to fix relationships damaged by COVID," in *USA Today*, https://archive.ph/KCoXq.
[471] Bullen, Paul and Onyx, Jenny (2005). "Measuring social capital in five communities in NSW," https://bit.ly/3NyY6mf.
[472] Australian Bureau of Statistics. Measuring Social Capital: An Australian Framework and Indicators, 2004, https://bit.ly/3yQShfT.

conditions, impairments and disabilities. Specifically, community participation (structural social capital) is indispensable to develop an effective community-based program to improve health and well-being of those with chronic health conditions or disabilities.[473]

While the loss of social capital from lockdowns is real and significant, I do not currently have access to reliable data to assess the magnitude of such harms.

14.2 Long-term impacts on immigration

Lockdowns and border closures have directly reduced migration to Australia in the short run. The ABS reported on 17 December 2021 that "There were more people departing from, than arriving into, Australia during the pandemic, reversing the historical migration pattern ... Australia recorded a net loss of 88,800 people in 2020-21."[474] A Grattan Institute report, *Migrants in the Workforce*, reported that about 1.5 million temporary migrants were in Australia's workforce as of January 2022, compared with almost 2 million in 2019.[475] On 13 May 2022, the *Financial Review* reported a "state of paralysis," with businesses stressed at the slowed immigration flow.[476]

By damaging the strength of and trust in our national institutions and leadership, Australian lockdowns may have created a longer-term loss of attractiveness of the country among migrants. Some Australian citizens born overseas have expressed on social media a commitment to permanently abandon Australia for freer countries, or have bad-mouthed Australia to their friends and relatives in the

---

[473] Lee, Jeong Kyu et al (2020). "Investigating the relationships between social capital, chronic health conditions and health status among Australian adults: findings from an Australian national cohort survey," in *BMC Public Health* volume 20, Article number: 329, https://archive.ph/jNkPC.

[474] Australian Bureau of Statistics. "More people emigrated from, than immigrated into, Australia in 2020-21," 17 December 2021, https://bit.ly/3wF8sLE.

[475] Mackey, Will et al (2020), "Australia is missing 500,000 migrants, but we don't need visa changes to lure them back," in *The Conversation*, 4 May 2022, https://archive.ph/pFQAr.

[476] Greber, Jacob et al (2022), "'State of paralysis'. Business despair over sluggish immigration flow," *Financial Review*, 13 May 2022, https://archive.ph/Hzk2X.

nations of their origin, thereby reducing the prospect of such people applying to migrate to Australia.[477]

Immigration is critical to a prosperous Australia. It is a key policy instrument for dealing with demographic and economic problems like the rapid ageing of Australia's population, falling birth rates, and the need for skilled labour. For example, since 1976, births per woman have been lower than 2.1 in Australia, which would lead to a shrinking population unless it is offset by net migration into the country. A geopolitical strategic argument can also be made that migration is necessary for Australia.

Immigration has many other impacts. The 2021 Intergenerational Report contains a detailed diagram[478] that illustrates the kinds of impacts that immigration has. As the report notes, "While the impact of migration can be estimated in economic measures such as GDP per person, broader quality-of-life impacts are more difficult to measure. For example, the contributions of migrants to cultural diversity, community connections or innovation are important but difficult to quantify … Migration should be kept at or below the capacity of the destination city or region to absorb new migrants, taking into account impacts on incumbent populations."[479]

Short-term benefits of lower immigration may include some domestic workers getting jobs or wage levels that they might not have otherwise gotten, but the longer-term harms to Australia of reduced intake of immigrants almost surely outweigh any such benefits.

Australian media have reported that "[e]conomists are divided on the future of immigration when international borders are re-opened with some warning more new arrivals will lead to lower wages and

---

[477] bdhSterling (2021). "Why the Border Closure has Prompted Many People to Leave Australia," 2 July 2021, https://archive.ph/ErnKH, "As a reaction to the severity of lockdown and what they see as the draconian closure of borders, a growing number of Australians are looking to leave permanently because of disillusionment at the action. Many of them are immigrants who have lived in Australia for some time."

[478] Treasurer of Australia, *2021 Intergenerational Report* (Figure 2.1, page 18), https://bit.ly/3LPIjhm.

[479] *Ibid*, p. 24.

fewer job opportunities for locals as others want population growth to bolster the nation's pandemic recovery."[480] I am among those economists who judge that lower net migration to Australia in 2020 and 2021, and in future years, would impose a significant net cost on Australia.

Migration is a decision based on the relative levels of freedom and opportunity in the host and source countries. With other nations from which Australian immigrants come such as India and China continuing to perform badly on key indicators of freedom, there is less reason to worry that the labour inflows into Australia will be permanent. Due to the challenge of assessing the likely duration of the immigration decline and its net effects on Australia, I do not include changes in immigration as part of the costs of lockdowns in this report.

14.3 Increase in non-homicide crime

Beyond homicides, covered previously, have lockdowns changed the levels of other crimes? With their energy diverted to the enforcement of public health orders, the police and courts have been distracted in 2020 and 2021 away from crimes of all types. This crowding-out is likely to have allowed many types of crimes to flourish below the surface, with longer-term impacts not yet understood.

Some evidence suggests that lockdowns have driven an increase in online child sex abuse. *The Australian* reported on 12 October 2020[481] that:

> Authorities are becoming increasingly concerned at the surge in child sex abuse, with the number of arrests and charges since the start of the coronavirus pandemic almost double that of the same period last year. "These type of offenders are using the lockdown restrictions to take advantage of vulnerable children who may be spending an

---

[480] *Sydney Morning Herald.* "Experts split on whether boosting migration helps or hinders economy," 7 August 2021, https://bit.ly/3LzI0Hy.

[481] Lewis, Rosie (2020). "Child sex predators rampant as Covid forces kids online," in *The Australian*, 12 October 2020, https://bit.ly/3lEl7YS.

increased amount of time online during this period," Mr Dutton said.

[T]here has been a 129 per cent increase in the number of reports of online child sex abuse material to the commissioner from March to August compared to the 2019 monthly average.

There have also been sporadic reports that crimes have increased in Australia during this period because police resources have been diverted to public health functions. For example:

I heard there has been a burglary boom in Brisbane. Police have told a mate that with all their attention on closing the QLD border, looking for burglars is a low priority.[482]

However, in the absence of reliable data at this time, I omit from my estimate of the costs of lockdowns any increase in non-homicide crime.

14.4 Environmental costs

In Section 8.4 I discussed the effects of lockdowns on CO_2 emissions, some of which may count as benefits and others as costs. I also mentioned the polluting effects of increased packaging requirements during lockdowns.

While these costs and benefits are important, in the absence of reliable data at this time and consistent with my analysis for the UK in *The Great Covid Panic*, I ignore environmental costs or benefits of lockdowns in this report.

---

[482] Tweet dated 25 October 2020 by Cameron Murray, https://bit.ly/3ly9cvT.

15. Summary of costs and benefits and conclusion

The analysis in this report confirms unequivocally that lockdowns and border closures have not advanced the "greater good." Rather, they have set back the greater good very significantly.

15.1 Summary

I summarise the findings of this CBA below.

15.1.1 *Benefits of lockdowns*

In this paper I calculate the following upper-end estimate for the total benefit of lockdowns:

9,951 (total COVID deaths averted) x 5 (healthy years lost per COVID death) x 6 (WELLBYs per QALY) x 1.02 (accommodating losses to long COVID) + 131 (non-COVID deaths averted) x 50 (healthy years lost per each such death) x 6 (WELLBYs per QALY) = **343,800 WELLBYs**, or **57,300 QALYs**, in all.

Dividing the total benefit of 343,800 WELLBYs by 24, we get approximately 14,325 WELLBYs saved per month during 2020 and 2021 by Australia's stop-start lockdowns and related policies.

15.1.2 *Costs*

Table 15.1 below summarises the costs of lockdowns in **WELLBYs per month** for Australia, with data sourced from the foregoing chapters of this report.

Category	Disrupted area	Costs in original units on average per month for 2020, 2021	Costs in WELLBYs on average per month for 2020, 2021	Costs beyond 2021
Lost GDP and increased expenditure	Economic loss	$8.045 billion per month	482,700 WELLBYs per month	
Lost Wellbeing	Lost well-being (life satisfaction)	Drop in life satisfaction of 0.2 on a 0-10 scale on average per year of stop-start lockdowns	428,334 WELLBYs per month	
	Non-COVID excess deaths in 2020 and 2021	7,940 additional non-COVID deaths from lockdowns in the first two years of the pandemic	9,937 WELLBYs per month	
Future costs	Reduction in the general lifespan of all Australians	Loss of one week of life for the average Australian		59,304 WELLBYs per year for the next 50 years
	Lost future productivity of children born during lockdowns	Lifetime earnings of 600,000 children born during 2020 and 2021 drops by $18 billion (or $30,000 per child) over a 35-year working life due to reduced IQ; a total WELLBY loss of 1,080,000 WELLBYs		30,857 WELLBYs per year starting in 20 years and continuing for the ensuing 35 years
	Lost future productivity of children of school age during lockdowns	$465 million in lost lifetime earnings of schoolchildren (27,900 WELLBYs over 35 years of working life)		797 WELLBYs per year (27900/35) starting in 10 years and continuing for the ensuing 35 years

Table 15.1: Summary of the estimated short-term and longer-term costs of Australia's lockdowns and border closures

The first three rows, showing estimates of costs paid during the lockdown period, average out to 920,971 WELLBYs per month, or 920,971 x 24 = **22.10 million WELLBYs in all over two years.**

The next three rows present the tally of future costs of the lockdowns implemented in 2020 and 2021 and are discounted in order to be comparable with other lockdown costs which are expressed in "2021 well-being currency." The present value of these future costs at a 5% yearly discount rate is **1.31 million WELLBYs.**

The sum of these two cost estimates, **23.41 million WELLBYs,** is the total estimated cost of lockdowns in 2021 well-being "currency."

The spreadsheet containing the net present value calculations underpinning these figures is available on the internet for public perusal.[483]

15.1.3 *Cost-benefit ratio*

Choosing conservatively to exclude or under-estimate many costs, and to make generous estimates of benefits, I estimate the maximum benefits from Australia's lockdown policies to be **343,800** WELLBYs, and the minimum costs from lockdowns to be **23.41** million WELL-BYs.

This indicates that **the costs of Australia's COVID lockdowns have been at least 68 times greater than the benefits they delivered.** Because I make assumptions in this CBA that are highly favourable to the government's choice to pursue a lockdown strategy, the true ratio of costs to benefits of the Australian COVID lockdowns is likely to be greater than this.

I conclude with five general observations that express my concerns about what has happened in Australia during this dark time, and include some suggestions for the future.

---

[483] http://sanjeev.sabhlokcity.com/Misc/Final-cost-table-CBA.xlsx.

15.2 Observation 1: The sacrifice of the young allegedly to protect the old

Australia's leadership seems not to have seriously considered the costs of lockdowns before imposing them in response to the modest threat posed by COVID. Governments have not demonstrated that their actions would yield maximum total welfare. Our governments owe the people a full costing of their lockdown policies that counts both whole lives cut short or extended (i.e., lives saved from COVID or taken for other reasons) and changes in the quality of life such as well-being, both in the short run and in the longer run.

The abandonment of their duty to promote the total welfare of society in the face of COVID has been seen in leaders in Australia and elsewhere. Politicians across the world have disproportionately valued death from COVID and undervalued all other kinds of deaths and suffering. They said, in effect, that dozens of deaths from cancer are worth one death from COVID. This grotesque reasoning has never been publicly articulated for obvious reasons.

Governments ignored the basic principles of policy making which were well-established in Western nations and in Australia. The rationality that was part of our inheritance from the Enlightenment was cast aside at the onset of the COVID era.

Even at the time of writing in mid-2022, we continually hear about the count of COVID cases rather than the count of people suffering symptoms or hospitalised with any of the various health threats that humans face. We know that "[a]pproximately 9% of the world's population is affected annually [with the flu], with up to 1 billion infections."[484] If we were to count the cases of all viruses that infect us and treat them like the fearsome pestilence of the sort that COVID has been elevated to in the media, we would do nothing all day but hide under the bed.

---

[484] Influenza Update (2011). *Pharmacy and Therapeutics*, v.36(10); 2011 Oct, https://www.ncbi.nlm.nih.gov/pmc/articles/PMC3278149/.

What matters is human suffering and death – not whether someone tests positive to a particular virus.

Children and young adults have become the human sacrifice offered by Australia's leadership on the altar of "saving Granny's life" – when in fact there was never any evidence of a connection in a COVID world between shelter-in-place orders and lives saved. As I have written elsewhere,[485] we have not witnessed in the COVID era the fight of our lives against a fearsome pestilence. We have instead seen politicians willingly sacrificing their people's welfare, hoping the people see their actions as a sufficient offering. It has been the modern analogue of killing virgins in the hope of getting a good harvest.

15.3 Observation 2: Why did our institutions cave in to groupthink?

We need to think hard about how our institutions in COVID times became the victim of groupthink.

In my book, *The Great Covid Panic*, my co-authors and I discuss a range of contributing factors, including those related to crowd psychology and the groupthink it creates, as part of our explanation for why the events since mid-March 2020 transpired as they did. In his 1841 book, *Extraordinary Popular Delusions and the Madness of Crowds*, Charles MacKay puts it well when he says:

> Men, it has been well said, think in herds; it will be seen that they go mad in herds, while they only recover their senses slowly, one by one.

Fear, which ran high in March 2020 and helped to form the COVID crowd and associated groupthink, is a very powerful emotion because it essentially shuts out focus on anything but the perceived threat. It is very effective in fight-or-flight scenarios where there really is a threat, but because of the intense focus that it creates, fear can cripple us when we are responding to something that is in reality not as big a threat as we imagine it to be.

---

[485] Foster, Gigi (2021). "Stop this human sacrifice: the case against lockdowns," *The Sydney Morning Herald*, 28 June 2021, https://archive.ph/L9RiM.

The US government in the time of the Great Depression tried to reduce fear in its population. FDR famously opined that 'The only thing we have to fear is fear itself' – and that statement is still applicable. Australia's governments were responsible in early 2020 to try to reduce fear so people could have responded to other things in their environment and participated in a healthy economy to the extent possible. If people are fearful, uncertain, and unsure what the future holds, they will be less likely to invest, less likely to spend, less likely to do everything that we know economic activity is based on, and that means that society – and the economy – will falter.

In my book, my co-authors and I have proposed some options for countering such mass-scale groupthink in the future. In his 2020 book, *The Great Hysteria and The Broken State*, Sanjeev Sabhlok has also offered his ideas for dealing with the underlying incentive problems that lock in groupthink inside governments.

15.4 Observation 3: The need to respect liberty

Lockdowns unambiguously breach the United Nations Universal Declaration of Human Rights, particularly Article 30:

> Nothing in this Declaration may be interpreted as implying for any State, group or person any right to engage in any activity or to perform any act aimed at the destruction of any of the rights and freedoms set forth herein.[486]

Police brutality in Australia reached a level during 2020 and 2021 where even international leaders commented adversely about what was occurring in Australia. We needed our governments to take actions to aggressively defend human rights in our collective hour of need, but the reverse happened. Shallow arguments have been used to overrule human rights. Those who have sought to defend human rights have been attacked both verbally and physically.

Many historical figures remind us of the need for great caution while breaching human rights – e.g.:

---

[486] United Nations. "Universal Declaration of Human Rights," https://archive.ph/MTCnt.

> Once a government is committed to the principle of silencing the voice of opposition, it has only one way to go, and that is down the path of increasingly repressive measures, until it becomes a source of terror to all its citizens and creates a country where everyone lives in fear."
>
> – Harry S. Truman

It is now overwhelmingly clear that the actions of many public health organisations across the world during the COVID pandemic have been totalitarian, if not criminal, with manifestly unethical behaviour on display from those in positions of power. On 14 May 2021, members of the Scientific Pandemic Influenza Group on Behaviour admitted to their use of 'unethical' methods during the pandemic and expressed regret.

> Members of the Scientific Pandemic Influenza Group on Behaviour (SPI-B) expressed regret about the tactics in a new book about the role of psychology in the Government's Covid-19 response.
>
> SPI-B warned in March last year that ministers needed to increase "the perceived level of personal threat" from Covid-19 because "a substantial number of people still do not feel sufficiently personally threatened".
>
> Gavin Morgan, a psychologist on the team, said: "Clearly, using fear as a means of control is not ethical. Using fear smacks of totalitarianism. It's not an ethical stance for any modern government."[487]

The discipline of public health has been severely tainted during this period. Both a reckoning and a rehabilitation of the public health discipline are needed in order to restore the public's trust in public health officials' and practitioners' ability to discharge their stated duties. Many behavioural scientists too, like so many other professional groups, have been complicit in the destruction wrought by the policies of this era and require significant internal re-evaluation of their ethical principles and priorities.

---

[487] *The Telegraph*. "Use of fear to control behaviour in Covid crisis was 'totalitarian', admit scientists," 14 May 2021, https://archive.ph/9yD8l.

15.5 Observation 4: What should governments have done? What should be done now?

I outlined many of my answers to these questions at the Victorian PAEC in 2020, but elaborate on them further below.

Follow the plan

Our pandemic response plans that were in place in March 2020 (including for COVID, such as the 10 March 2020 Victorian pandemic plan specifically for COVID) embedded the logic that there could be no gain from blanket lockdowns. These plans were summarily scrapped in mid-March 2020. Our governments should have followed these plans. They should have controlled fear, directed resources and attention towards protecting the most vulnerable, set policy based on the knowledge of a range of experts including economists rather than only health scientists, and evaluated the likely impact of their policy choices on total human welfare as time progressed and more data became available.

Engage in public conversation and direct resources to those most in need

A public discussion should have been had when the pandemic first emerged about how most effectively to direct the resources we have towards people who are most likely to get serious symptoms or die from this virus if they contract it. Amassing and disseminating knowledge about how to protect vulnerable people, such as those in old-age homes – how to make their close contacts aware of the risks, and how to help them to best to protect themselves and others – is where our resources should have gone. Options for effective early treatment and prophylaxis should have been fully investigated at every stage as the situation developed and knowledge grew.

The government should have allowed those who are least likely to suffer the most severe consequences of COVID to get on with their lives. Others could have opted for protections suited to their perceived level of risk, including taking the vaccine. However, requiring vaccination with no regard to prior natural immunity as a pre-condition for travel, work, study, or social acceptance is not only scientifically illogical but violates human rights and bodily autonomy. Moreover, the COVID vaccines were never magic bullets: mass vaccination in Australia in 2021 failed to prevent more than 8,000 COVID deaths in the first half of 2022 alone.

While directly supporting the vulnerable, we should have learned from the mistakes of Sweden in the early stages of the pandemic and set high-risk individuals up on videoconference technology and other support to remain connected to family, friends, and communities. We could have subsidised immune-system support and work alternatives for high-risk groups, and targeted testing and monitoring towards aged-care workers and carers of high-risk individuals. We could have soaked up some of those who are now unemployed into the health sector to assist with these efforts. In fact, we have been doing the opposite, by ejecting experienced people from the health care sector for reasons not grounded in logic, morality, or science.

Provide income support that is targeted, limited and honest

Conditional on lockdowns, I supported the government's provision of income support, like JobKeeper for example, but only temporarily and only where it was absolutely necessary. Yet claiming that somehow those provisions were equivalent to fixing the fundamental problem, which is that our economy was stabbed in the stomach by our government, is facile. Lockdowns and JobKeeper never comprised a long-term solution to COVID, and programs like JobKeeper and increased funding for mental health support treated the symptoms rather than treating the disease itself, where the disease is one that we inflicted upon ourselves with lockdowns. Giving people money stems a bit of suffering in the short run but it does not solve the problem in the long run, so we were still left with massive costs of wholesale lockdowns for which the solution was simply to stop the lockdowns and get the economy moving again while offering thoughtful, creative, and targeted assistance for vulnerable people.

Evidence has emerged indicating that JobKeeper effected the transfer of vast amounts of taxpayer funds to people who did not need them. The pandemic plans of Australia did not have any provision for lockdowns, which is why the Treasury and our annual budgets had no contingency plan for a scheme like JobKeeper. As one might expect, such a policy crafted 'on the run' was far from perfect. A full examination of its problems is beyond the scope of this report, but indicative evidence is quoted below.

There were three key flaws in the scheme. These flaws led to a record bonanza in corporate profits, payouts to shareholders, both offshore and domestic, and executive bonuses:

- There was no "clawback" mechanism in JobKeeper which ensured subsidies would be paid back by those rorting it,
- Subsidiaries of multinational companies were allowed to claim it,
- The list of JobKeeper recipients was kept a secret from the start, and remains a secret, in contrast to similar corporate welfare schemes in New Zealand, the US and elsewhere.[488]

15.6 Observation 5: An alternative government script

If the government wishes to do the right thing, even today, it will need a new pragmatic script that calms people down. The script could look something like this (taken from my August 2020 testimony to Victoria's PAEC):

> Covid is like a particularly severe flu and a bit more infectious. It has been added to what is circulating in humanity. We can't stop the virus from spreading, and we don't want to. The sooner it moves across the general population, the sooner it will run out of carriers and come to a halt on its own – through a combination of factors such as the development of antibodies, existing T-cell immunity, and heterogeneous susceptibility across individuals.

---

[488] *Michael West Media.* "Business whispers: how Treasurer Josh Frydenberg squandered $40bn on JobKeeper," 16 October 2021, https://archive.ph/JKqKt.

Most of us will be unaffected by the virus and unaware of any infection. Each of us should do what supports our health, happiness, and immune system. If we get seriously ill, we should go to hospital. Otherwise, get on with our life.

We are in a privileged position in Australia to be able to learn how best to combat this virus, and it is to target assistance to the areas that are most vulnerable in the community while allowing other people to get back to work and back to study.

In sum, lockdowns were a colossal mistake. Suppression of COVID has led to the loss of vastly more of human life-years from non-COVID causes. Attempts to shield the general population were ultimately futile, causing misery for no long-term gain, and preventing immunity from emerging. In future pandemics, we must not punish the healthy and put our economies into a coma, but rather focus our attention and protection on the people in our population who are most vulnerable to serious effects of the threat.

Moving forward, we need to secure medicines and establish treatment protocols that work to reduce the severity of COVID symptoms, while dropping all restrictions on freedoms in the name of COVID and pledging never again to betray Australia by re-imposing them.

www.ingramcontent.com/pod-product-compliance
Lightning Source LLC
Chambersburg PA
CBHW061245220326
41599CB00028B/5539